CONTACT DERMATITIS

Edited by **Young Suck Ro**

Contact Dermatitis
Edited by Young Suck Ro

Published by InTech
Janeza Trdine 9, 51000 Rijeka, Croatia

Publishing Process Manager Bojana Zelenika

Technical Editor Teodora Smiljanic

Cover Designer InTech Design Team

Additional hard copies can be obtained from orders@intechopen.com

Contact Dermatitis, Edited by Young Suck Ro
p. cm.
ISBN 978-953-307-577-8

For EU product safety concerns:
IN TECH d.o.o., Prolaz Marije Krucifikse Kozulić 3, 51000 Rijeka, Croatia,
info@intechopen.com or visit our website at intechopen.com.

Meet the editor

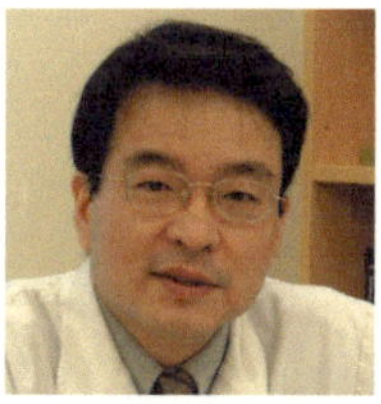

Having obtained his doctorate from Hanyang University, Korea in 1981, Professor Young Suck Ro began his career working for Department of Dermatology of said university and has since progressed to become Head of Department. In a career spanning some thirty years, he has achieved a number of notable accolades, including being award the British Conference Fellowship Award (1991) presented by the British Association of Dermatologists; Pacific Research of Korean Award (1991), and the Hanmi Research of Contact Dermatitis Award both presented by Korean Dermatological Association (2005).

Contents

Preface

We are proud to present the first book on *Contact Dermatitis*, which was written to reflect the current state of the science, practice, and art of dermatology. In this book, we have invited a number of skilled individuals to share their expertise with our readers. *Contact Dermatitis* is an excellent tool to be utilized for anyone who requires help in diagnosing patients with a conundrum or treating patients with a therapeutically challenging dermatitis.

During the last decade, our insight into the knowledge of pathogenesis has increased. Diagnostic modalities have been modified and newly developed. Our aim is to encourage the understanding of scientific aspects of dermatology, and to provide an updated reference guide to contact dermatitis. A distinct feature of this book is that it describes numerous possible allergens causing contact dermatitis, and extensive details of research in the basic sciences and advanced diagnostic techniques are provided. Thus, this book will help our readers understand more about contact dermatitis. It is our hope that this book will assist physicians in treating contact dermatitis in the best way possible. Most importantly, we hope that this text will benefit patients in the future.

We thank all authors. We would also like to thank the production team of InTech for their efforts throughout the preparation of this book.

Prof. Dr. Young Suck Ro
Head Professor and Chairman, Department of Dermatology,
Hanyang University Hospital, Seoul,
Korea

Part 1

Epidemiology

1

Epidemiology of Contact Dermatitis

Jesús Jurado-Palomo[1], Álvaro Moreno-Ancillo[1], Irina Diana Bobolea[2],
Carmen Panizo Bravo[1] and Iván Cervigón González[3]
[1]*Department of Allergology, Nuestra Señora del Prado General Hospital,*
Talavera de la Reina,
[2]*Department of Allergology, University Hospital La Paz, Madrid*
[3]*Department of Dermatology, Nuestra Señora del Prado General Hospital,*
Talavera de la Reina
Spain

1. Introduction

Substances that are responsible of contact dermatitis can be irritant, as chemical or physical agents that causes irritant contact dermatitis (ICD) , or sensitizers, when causes a tissue inflammation damage with allergic mechanism (allergic contact dermatitis or ACD). ICD results from contacts with irritant substances, while ACD is a delayed-type immunological reaction in response to contact with an allergen in sensitized individuals. Primary lesions of occupational contact dermatitis (OCD) are usually found at the site of contact with the irritant or allergen; in the case of ACD, secondary lesions may occur subsequently on other sites of the body that have never been in contact with the allergens (Meneghini & Angelini, 1984).

Contact dermatitis is a common inflammatory skin disease in industrialized countries, with a great socioeconomic impact. It is one of the most common occupational diseases (Coenreaads & Goncalo, 2007; Saint-Mezard et al 2004). Epidemiology is also used to analyse whether it is more common in specific groups, and which factors are associated with the occurrence of contact dermatitis (or its subtypes) in specific populations or subgroups.

2. Factors contributing to contact dermatitis

Studies have been investigated a possible association between different factors and contact sensitization.

2.1 Gender and age

Women are usually more frequently patch-tested, and have more positivity results than men (García-Gavín et al, 2011). Gender differences may be attributed to social and environmental factors; females are more likely to have nickel sensitivity because of increased wearing of jewellery, and males are more likely to have chromate sensitivity from occupational exposure (Ruff & Besilto, 2006).

Rui et al estimate the prevalence of nickel, cobalt and chromate allergy in a population of consecutive patients and investigate the possible association with individual and occupational risk factors (Rui et al, 2010). This study showed interesting associations between some occupations and nickel, chromate and cobalt allergy.

ACD in children, until recently, was considered rare (Hammonds et al, 2009). One of the largest population-based patch test studies of unselected pediatric patients, which also provides specific relevance information, found the prevalence of past or current relevant reactions to be 7%, with a higher risk seen in females (Mortz et al, 2002). This is considerably lower than the prevalence in selected pediatric populations (symptomatic patients). Nickel is the most common sensitizer in almost all studies pertaining to pediatric contact dermatitis. Thus, the real prevalence of ACD (defined as a positive patch test with clinical correlation with the dermatitis experienced by a symptomatic individual) ranges from 14% to 77% among children referred for patch testing due to clinical suspicion of contact dermatitis (Bruckner et al, 2000; Fernández Vozmediano & Armario Hita, 2005; Seidenari et al, 2005; Lewis et al, 2004).

Eczema in adults usually exists for years, compromising quality of life and occupational choices. The flexural areas, shoulders, head-and-neck, and hands are typically affected in 5-15% of cases (Katsarou et al, 2001). The relationship between atopy and contact allergy remains unclear. Atopic dermatitis is a risk factor for allergic contact sensitization (Dotterud & Smith-Sivertsen, 2007). ACD increases with age in atopics (Lammintausta et al, 1992).

Contact dermatitis is a significant health problem affecting the elderly people. Impaired epidermal barrier function and delayed cutaneous recovery after injury enhances susceptibility to both irritants and allergens. Exposure to more numerous potential sensitizers and for greater durations influences the rate of allergic contact dermatitis in this population. Medical co-morbidities, including stasis dermatitis and venous ulcerations, further exacerbate this clinical picture (Prakash & Davis, 2010). Aging is correlated with the rate and type of contact sensitization, but only a few studies have evaluated patch test reactivity in elderly individuals with an adequately large population (Nedorost & Stevens, 2001; Balato et al, 2011).

2.2 Race

Black people may be less susceptible to sensitisation by weaker allergens and have a lower incidence of ICD because of greater compaction of the lipid component of the stratum corneum, conferring improved barrier function (Robinson, 1999; Astner et al, 2006). Ethnicity is a possible endogenous factor implicated in ICD. While there is a clinical consensus that blacks are less reactive and Asians are more reactive than Caucasians, the data supporting this hypothesis rarely reaches statistical significance. Modjtahedi SP et al conclude that race could be a factor in ICD, which has practical consequences regarding topical product testing requirements, an ever-expanding global market, occupational risk assessment, and the clinical thinking about ICD (Modjtahedi & Maibach, 2002).

2.3 Exposure to irritants and allergens

The most important risk factor for OCD is the exposure to irritants. Well-known irritants are water (wet work), detergents and cleansing agents, hand cleaners, chemicals, cutting fluids, and abrasives. ACD is a common skin condition that can be difficult to diagnose without the aid of a specific diagnostic tool called patch testing. Patch testing performed with a relevant panel of contact allergens is the ultimate confirmatory test of ACD (see Chapter titled "Allergens (patch test studies) from the European Baseline Series" on this book). Correctly identifying the inciting allergen permits appropriate personal avoidance.

2.4 Personal history of atopic dermatitis

General population studies have repeatedly found that atopic dermatitis is the most important risk factor for hand eczema (Meding & Swanbeck, 1990; Dotterud & Falk, 1995; Yngveson M et al, 2000; Mortz et al, 2001; Meding & Jarvholm, 2002; Bryld et al, 2003; Josefson et al, 2006). Thus, the effect of atopic dermatitis seemed to level off with increasing age. Whether association between hand eczema on the one hand and atopic dermatitis or atopy on the other hand is explained by null mutations in the filaggrin gene (de Jongh et al, 2008; Carlsen et al, 2011), by an altered immune response (Davis et al, 2010; McFadden et al, 2011), or by their combination is currently unknown. Future studies should aim to investigate the distribution of these risk factors.

2.5 Other possible association

Studies have re-investigated a possible association between these lifestyle factors (alcohol drinking and tobacco smoking) and contact sensitization (Thyssen et al, 2010).

2.6 Analyzed literature

A substantial number of studies have also investigated the prevalence of contact allergy in the general population and in unselected subgroups of the general population (Thyssen et al, 2007). These studies have demonstrated variations in the prevalence of contact allergy depending on the selected study population and year of investigation. These studies are of high value as they tend to be less biased than studies using clinical populations and as they are important for health care decision makers when they allocate resources. Literature was examined using Pubmed-Medline, Biosis, Science Citation Index, and dermatology text books. Search terms included hand eczema, hand dermatitis, general population, unselected, healthy, prevalence, incidence, risk factor, and epidemiology. In observational studies on contact dermatitis, the ascertainment of cases varied from intensive efforts by a medical examination of the complete study population to the relatively easy-to-apply method of self-administered questionnaires; or by a combination of both. However, a diagnosis of contact dermatitis based on a self-administered questionnaire is significantly less valid than the diagnosis based on examination by a dermatologist (McCurdy et al, 1989).

3. Hand eczema in the general population

Information on the prevalence of hand eczema, contact sensitivity and contact dermatitis in the general population can be obtained from cross-sectional studies that were performed recently (Thyssen et al, 2009; Nielsen et al, 2001a, 2001b; Mortz et al, 2001;

Sosted et al, 2005; Lerbaek et al, 2007). Several studies have investigated the incidence of hand eczema in the general population (Bo et al, 2008; Hald et al, 2008; Moberg et al, 2009; Lind et al, 2007).

Hand eczema is the most frequent occupational skin disease. In many jobs the skin on the hands is subjected to damage caused by contact with skin irritants and contact allergens. Several studies have investigated the incidence and prevalence of hand eczema in the general population.

3.1 Usefulness of patch testing

Patch testing remains the gold standard for the diagnosis of ACD (Devos & Van Der Valk, 2002; Uter W et al, 2009). Quality control of patch testing is both a prerequisite for, and an objective of, clinical epidemiology of contact dermatitis. Continuous development of test standards concerning the composition of test series, test concentration, and vehicle and standardization of test readings is provided by the national and international research groups on contact dermatitis.

Many studies in contact dermatitis are based on populations that have been patch tested; usually this means that the participants visited a clinic or a hospital for being evaluated on having contact dermatitis. There are a variety of types of irritant reactions - some can look identical to allergic reactions. The recognised convention for recording patch test reactions is as follows:

+/− doubtful:	faint erythema only
+ weak:	erythema, maybe papules
++ strong:	vesicles, infiltration
+++ extreme:	bullous
IR:	irritant

3.2 Measures of disease frequency (incidence and prevalence)

The epidemiologist deals with necessity of data on defined populations. The most basic setting giving rise to epidemiological data is the evaluation of the occurrence of a disease in the presence of an exposure. The exposure may be present or absent and the disease may be present or absent.

Measures of disease frequencies include *prevalence*, which is the amount of disease that is already present in a population; *incidence*, which refers to the number of new cases of contact dermatitis during a defined period in a specified population; and "incidence rate" (IR), which is the number of non-diseased persons who become diseased within a certain period of time, divided by the number of person-years in the population. All measures of disease frequency consist of the number of cases as the numerator, and the size of the population under study as the denominator. Sensitivity and specificity of the diagnostic instruments used are important. In epidemiological studies, an overestimation of prevalence can result from low sensitivity/specificity.

The three most important types of observational study in the epidemiology of contact dermatitis are follow up studies, case-control studies and cross-sectional studies. In follow-up studies, selection of subjects is based upon exposure to the factor of interest. Instead of exposure, the presence or absence of a risk factor (e.g. nickel allergy, or atopy) can also be chosen as basis for comparison. In case-control studies, the subjects are selected according to their disease status. Information on the past exposure of the persons with contact dermatitis (cases) and the non-diseased persons (controls) is collected. In cross-sectional studies, a study population is selected regardless of exposure status or disease status (in contrast to case-control and follow-up studies).

Data on the incidence and prevalence of occupational dermatoses are scarce. The most important sources of data are occupational disease registries, case series of patients visiting dermatology clinics, and a limited number of cross-sectional studies in one or more occupational groups.

3.3 Incidence and prevalence of contact dermatitis and contact sensitisation

Incidence of hand eczema: Several studies have investigated the incidence of hand eczema in the general population (Lantinga et al, 1984; Yngveson M, 2000; Meding & Jarvholm, 2004; Brisman J et al, 1998; Meding et al, 2006; Lind, 2007; Lerbaek et al, 2007). The median incidence rate was 5.5 cases/1000 person-years (range 3.3–8.8). Stratified by sex, the median incidence rate of hand eczema was 9.6 cases/1000 person-years (range 4.6–11.4) among women and 4.0 cases/1000 person-years (range 1.4–7.4) among men (Thyssen et al, 2010).

Prevalence of hand eczema: Few studies showed that the 1-year median prevalence of hand eczema in the general population was 9.7% (11.4% among women and 5.4% among men) and that the 1-year weighted average prevalence was 9.1% (10.5% among women and 6.4% among men) (Lantinga et al, 1984; Agrup, 1969; Peltonen, 1979; Menné et al, 1982; Kavli & Forde, 1984; Meding, 1990; Meding & Swanbeck, 1987; Meding & Jarvholm, 2002; Ortengren, 1999; Meding et al, 2001; Brisman J et al, 1998; Montnemery et al, 2005; Bo et al, 2008; Fowler et al, 2006; Hald et al, 2008; Svedman et al, 2007; Lind et al, 2007).

Population studies may give valuable information on the magnitude of the disease problem. Different data was found when compared the frequencies of positive path-tests reactions in the general population and in eczema patients at a dermatological clinic in the same area (Menné & Knudsen 1997) (Table 1). Publications based on data of patients visiting dermatology clinics and/or patch testing units can not be used to directly derive population related incidence or prevalence estimates. Data from incidence studies may support and direct strategies for the prevention of contact allergy and ACD, supporting conclusions derived from clinical surveillance data.

Nickel sulphate is the most common allergen in the standard series and the most common cause of allergic contact dermatitis, particularly in women. This gender difference is traditionally explained by increased exposure in women, due to direct skin contact with nickel-releasing metal, such as in jewellery, wristwatches, and clothing accessories. A possible association between nickel allergy and hand eczema in women has been addressed and supported by several population-based studies, whereas an association has been questioned in men (Nielsen et al, 2002; Peltonen, 1979; Meijer et al, 1995) (Tables 2 and 3).

Test substances	General population % positive of tested			Dermatological clinic % positive of tested		
	Men n=279	Women n=288	Total n=567	Men n= 262	Women n= 416	Total n= 672
Potassium dichromate	0.7	0.3	0.5	1.9	2.7	2.4
Neomycin sulfate	0.0	0.0	0.0	3.4	3.7	3.6
Thiuram mix	0.7	0.3	0.5	4.6	2.7	3.4
p-phenylenediamine	0.0	0.0	0.0	1.9	2.7	2.4
Cobalt chloride	0.7	1.4	1.1	2.3	2.7	2.5
Benzocaine	-	-	NT	0.4	0.7	0.6
Caine mix	0.0	0.0	0.0	-	-	NT
Formaldehyde	-	-	NT	1.9	2.2	2.1
Colophony (colophonium)	0.4	1.0	0.7	4.6	5.4	5.1
Quinoline mix	0.4	0.3	0.4	1.9	0.5	1.0
Balsam of Peru (*Myroxylon pereirae*)	0.7	1.4	1.1	3.4	5.4	4.6
N-isopropyl-N-phenyl-para-phenylenediamine (IPPD)	0.4	0.0	0.2	1.2	0.0	0.5
Wool alcohols (lanolin alcohol)	0.4	0.0	0.2	1.2	1.7	1.5
Mercapto mix	0.7	0.0	0.4	1.2	0.2	0.6
Epoxy resin	0.4	0.7	0.5	0.8	0.2	0.5
Paraben mix	0.4	0.3	0.4	0.8	0.2	0.5
para-Tertiary-butylphenol-formaldehyde resin (PTBP resin)	1.1	1.0	1.1	0.4	1.2	0.9
Fragrance mix	1.1	1.0	1.1	6.1	7.1	6.7
Ethyenediamine dihydrochloride	0.4	0.0	0.2	0.8	0.2	0.7
Quaternium-15	0.4	0.0	0.2	0.0	0.0	0.7
Nickel sulfate	2.2	11.1	6.7	4.2	16.1	11.0
Cl+Me-isothiazolinonec	0.4	1.0	0.7	0.4	0.7	0.6
Mercaptobenzothiazole	0.4	0.0	0.2	1.2	0.2	0.6
Primin	-	-	NT	0.4	1.5	1.0
Thiomersal	3.6	3.1	3.4	-	-	NT
Carba mix	0.7	0.0	0.4	-	-	NT

Table 1. Comparison of frequencies of positive patch-test reactions in the general population and in eczema at a dermatological clinic in the same area of greater Copenhagen in 1990 (Menné & Knudsen 1997).

Study	*N*	Allergens used for patch testing	Positive reaction to nickel; total (%)	Three most common allergens
Nielsen et al, 1992	567	TRUE-tests	6.7	Nickel, thimerosal, cobalt/Balsam of Peru
Nielsen et al, 1998	469	TRUE-tests	10.8	Nickel, fragance mix, and thimerosal
Schäfer et al, 2001	1141	Standard series	9.9	Nickel, fragance mix, and thimerosal
Akasya-Hillenbrand, 2002	542	Standard series	19.1	Nickel, potassium dichromate, and palladium chloride
Lazarov, 2006	2156	TRUE-tests	13.9	Nickel, fragrance mix, and potassium dichromate
Dotterud & Smith-Sivertsen, 2007	1236	TRUE-tests	17.6	Nickel, cobalt, and thimerosal
García-Gavín et al, 2011	1161	Spanish standard series	25.8	Nickel, potassium dichromate, and cobalt chloride

Table 2. Studies on contact dermatitis in the general population (list is not extensive).

Study	*n*	Allergens used for patch testing	Positive reaction to nickel; total (%)	Three most common allergens
Röckl et al, 1966	357	Not given; MCl/MI and PPD	2.5	Chromium, $HgCl_2$, and formaldehyde
Weston et al, 1986	314	Standard series	7.6	Neomycin, nickel, and chromium
Barros et al, 1991	562	Standard series	0.9	Neomycin, thimerosal, p-tertiary-butylphenol-formaldehide
Dotterud & Falk, 1994	424	Epiquick test	14.9	Nickel, cobalt, and MCl/MI
Mortz et al, 2001	1146	TRUE-tests	8.6	Nickel, fragance mix, and thimerosal/colophony/cobalt

Table 3. Studies on contact dermatitis in children (general population) (list is not extensive).

3.4 Current view on the spectrum of contact allergy to important sensitizers across Spain

In 2005, the Spanish Society of Allergology and Clinical Immunology (Sociedad Española de Alergología e Inmunología Clínica (SEAIC) in collaboration with the Allergy and

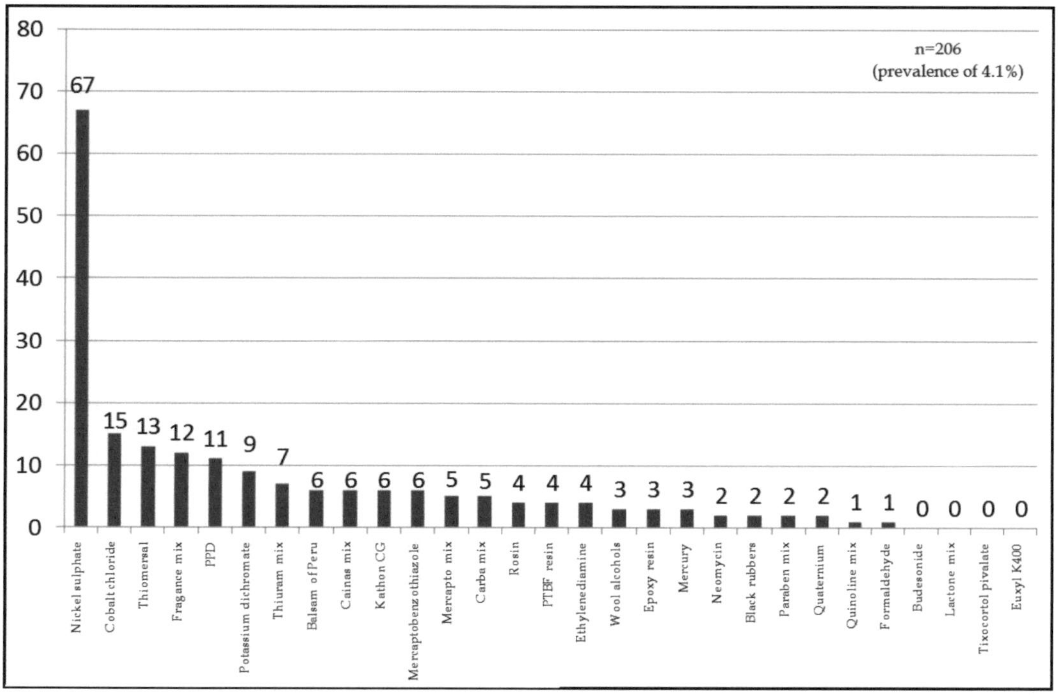

Fig. 1. Etiologic agents for contact dermatitis in *Alergológica*-2005.

Immunology Laboratory Abelló undertook the "Alergológica 2005" study with the aim of obtaining epidemiologic, clinical and socioeconomic information on allergic patients seen and treated by Allergology specialists in Spain.

In the particular case of contact dermatitis, the results from epicutaneous tests from the standard Spanish series for contact dermatitis were recorded by taking readings at 48 and 96 hours, and evaluating erythema-infiltration, papules and vesicles. Two hundred-six cases of contact dermatitis were diagnosed, which represents a prevalence of 4.1%. The mean age of the patients was 42.5 years and females clearly outnumbered men (2.5:1). In the etiology of contact dermatitis (Figure 1), the leading causes were metals, nickel and cobalt, together with chromium, with a total of 91 cases. Thiomersal is in third place with 13 cases, which represents 6.2% of all causes (Muñoz-Lejarazu, 2009).

3.5 Current view on the spectrum of contact allergy to important sensitizers across Europe

In 1996 a European surveillance network was created to analyze routinely collected data in various contact allergy units in several European countries (European Surveillance System on Contact Allergies [ESSCA]; www.essca-dc.org). ESSCA has been fully operational since 2001, with several surveillance networks currently participating, among them the British Contact Dermatitis Group; the IVDK in Germany, Switzerland, and Austria; the Northeast Italian Contact Dermatitis Group; and, more recently, the 5 hospital dermatology departments affiliated with the Spanish Group for Research Into Contact Dermatitis and Skin Allergy/Spanish Surveillance System on Contact Allergies (Hospital del Mar, Barcelona; Hospital La Princesa, Madrid; University General Hospital, Alicante; Complexo Hospitalario Universitario, Santiago de Compostela; and University Hospital Puerto Real) (García-Gavín et al, 2011). Nickel sulphate remains the most common allergen with standardized prevalences ranging from 19.7% (central Europe) to 24.4% (southern Europe). While a number of allergens shows limited variation across the four regions, such as

1.	Contact allergy was independent of enhanced IgE responsiveness.
2.	The median prevalence of contact allergy was 20% (adults 15–69 years).
3.	Contact allergy to a wide range of allergens as well as multiple contact allergy was observed in both children and adults.
4.	Contact allergy was most commonly observed against nickel, fragrances, and thimerosal.
5.	The proportion of nickel allergy out of contact allergy to at least 1 allergen has been increasing significantly over the past 4 decades.
6.	The median prevalence of nickel allergy among women was 17.1%.
7.	A median prevalence of 81.5% women, have pierced ears.
8.	Pierced ears are a strong risk factor for nickel allergy.
9.	Nickel contact allergy may be associated with hand eczema in women.
10.	Heavy smoking may be a risk factor for nickel allergy.

Table 4. Main findings from epidemiological population-based studies (published between 1966 and 2007) investigating contact allergy in the general population or subgroups of the general population (Thyssen et al, 2007).

Myroxylon pereirae (5.3-6.8%), cobalt chloride (6.2-8.8%) or thiuram mix (1.7-2.4%), the differences observed with other allergens may hint on underlying differences in exposures, for example: dichromate 2.4% in the UK (west) versus 4.5-5.9% in the remaining EU regions, methylchloroisothiazolinone/methylisothiazolinone 4.1% in the South versus 2.1-2.7% in the remaining regions (Uter et al, 2009).

The continuous collection and analysis of data within multicenter clinical epidemiology offer practical findings. Thyssen et al (2007) described main findings from epidemiological population-based studies (Table 2) investigating contact allergy in the general population or subgroups of the general population.

4. Occupational contact dermatitis

Work-related dermatoses, in particular hand dermatitis, are still among the most prevalent occupational diseases. Understanding the epidemiology of OCD is essential to determine etiologic factors of the disease and to make recommendations for its prevention.

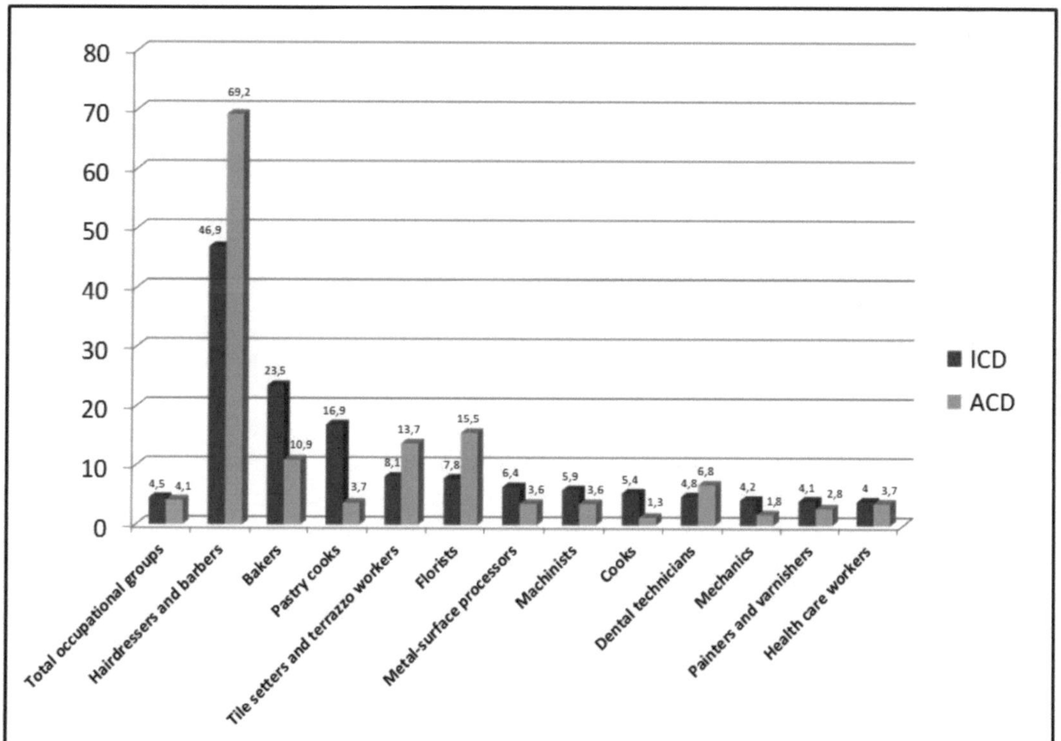

Incidence rates (per 10,000 employees) in the occupational groups with the highest risk for occupational skin diseases

Fig. 2. Incidence rates of ICD and ACD in the occupational groups with the highest risk for occupational skin diseases (Diepgen & Coenraads PJ, 2000).

Different professions have differing risks for occupational skin disease. Those at the highest risk for a contact dermatitis are hairdressers (yearly rate 120/100,000), printers (rate

71/100,000), machine tool operatives (rate 56/100,000), chemical/petroleum plant operatives (rate 45/100,000), assemblers (rate 35/100,000), and machine tool setters (rate 34/100,000) (Cherry et al, 2000). Accurate estimates of the incidence of occupational skin disease are difficult to find but a recent report from the EPIDERM and OPRA occupational skin disease surveillance project suggests a rate of 13 per 100 000 per year 5 and a prevalence of 15 per 10,000 of those ever employed has been quoted (Cherry et al, 2000).

Occupational disease registries provide national incidence data based on the notification of occupational skin diseases and are available in many countries. Although the comparison of national data are hampered by differences across countries in reporting and the definition of occupational diseases, the average incidence rate of registered occupational contact dermatitis in some countries lies around 0.5-1.9 cases per 1,000 full-time workers per year (Dickel et al, 2002; Halkier-Sorensen, 1996). The highest incidence rates were seen in hairdressers (Diepgen et al, 2000). In Figure 2, the incidence rates of ICD and ACD of employees of the twelve groups with the highest risk for an occupational skin disease are presented.

4.1 OCD in different work forces

The majority of work-related dermatoses, in particular hand dermatitis, comprise contact dermatitis (90-95%); the rest are of other dermatoses such as contact urticaria, oil acne, chloracne, chemically-induced leucoderma, and infections. In this section, different "work-related OCD" are discussed.

Health care workers (especially nurses) are often affected by OCD, whose "occupational sensitization pattern" comprises thiuram (rubber compounds), thiomersal (vaccine preservative) and several biocides (glutaraldehyde, formaldehyde, glyoxal and benzalkonium chloride) (Schnuch A et al, 1998). Operating-room staff is a subset of health-care workers (preparation and clean up may involve exposure to cleaning and disinfecting agents, and some workers may also have exposure to sterilizing agents, such as glutaraldehyde, and some workers may use ethylene oxide).

The frequency of OCD **in dental personnel** (dentists, dental assistants, dental technicians and orthodontics) has steadily increased over the last decades and currently considered to be about 40% (Uveges et al, 1995).

Hand eczema is a well-known and potentially severe drawback to the **hairdressing profession**. Hair cosmetic producers provide the hairdresser with a great variety of chemicals to fulfil stylist and customer desires. Smit et al studied a cohort of apprentice hairdressers (n=74) and nurses (n=111) and found an average incidence rate of hand dermatitis of 32.8 cases/100 person-years for the hairdressers, compared with 14.5 cases/100 person-years for the nurses (Smit et al, 1994).

Construction workers (bricklayers, manufacturers of concrete elements…) are in contact with wet cement products in the form of mortar or concrete. ACD due to hexavalent chromium in cement is still the most important contact allergy. Also, other substances have been identified (e.g., cobalt, tuber additives, epoxy resin, hexamenthylendiamine and isophorondiamine) (Geier & Struppek, 1995).

Metal workers are exposed to numerous exogenous factors that play a substantial role in the development of ACD as well as ICD. Even though nickel is regarded as the most frequent source of all reported metal allergies, metal-work fluids are the most important cause of irritant hand dermatitis (also exposed to other chemical irritants, such as cleaning detergents, solvents and degreasers) (Itschner L et al, 1996). Metal polishers remove excess metal and surface defects from various items such as the accessory parts of cars. The most commonly polished metals are aluminium, brass, bronze and zinc (Adams 1999).

4.2 Social and economic impact of contact dermatitis

The total economic impact of OCD is high according to the following costs (Diepgen & Coenrads, 2000):

- Direct costs of medical care, workers compensation or disability payments.
- Indirect costs associated with lost workdays and loss of productivity.
- Costs of occupational retraining.
- Costs attributable to the effects on the quality of life.

5. Conclusion

Numerous studies have investigated the prevalence and risk factors of hand eczema in the general population. Contact sensitization has become a significant public health problem. In many parts of the world, more than 20% of the adult population is suffering from contact allergy. The profile of sensitizations may differ in each country. However, nickel sulphate is the most prevalent allergen practically everywhere. Patch testing remains the gold standard for the diagnosis of ACD. Quality control of patch testing is both a prerequisite for, and an objective of, clinical epidemiology of contact dermatitis. Publications based on data of patients visiting dermatology clinics and/or patch testing units cannot be used to directly derive population related incidence or prevalence estimates.

6. Acknowledgment

We would like to thank the following individuals and associations for their collaboration, teaching and daily efforts, as well as for the material provided: the European Society of Contact Dermatitis (ESCD), the Dermatology Workgroup of the European Academy of Allergy and Clinical Immunology (EAACI), the Skin Allergy Committee of the Spanish Society of Allergology and Clinical Immunology (SEAIC), especially Dr. Pilar Iriarte Sotés (Arquitecto Marcide - Profesor Novoa Santos Hospital Complex, Ferrol, Spain); and the Spanish Workgroup on Contact Dermatitis (GEIDC) of the Spanish Academy of Dermatology and Venereology (AEDV). Their final input was crucial for the preparation of this manuscript.

7. References

Adams RM (1990). Metal polishers. In: Adams RM (ed) Occupational skin disease, 2nd ed; Saunders, Philadelphia, pp 638-639, ISBN 0-7216-2926-1.

Agrup G (1969). Hand eczema and other hand dermatosis in South Sweden. *Acta Derm Venereol,* Vol 49, (Suppl. 61): 1–91, ISSN 0001-5555.

Akasya-Hillenbrand E, Ozkaya-Bayazit E (2002). Patch test results in 542 patients with suspected contact dermatitis in Turkey. *Contact Dermatitis,* Vol.46, No.1 (January 2002), pp. 17-23, ISSN 0105-1873

Astner S, Burnett N, Rius-Díaz F, Doukas AG, González S, González E (2006). Irritant contact dermatitis induced by a common household irritant: a noninvasive evaluation of ethnic variability in skin response. *J Am Acad Dermatol,* Vol.54. No.3 (March 2006), pp. 458-465, ISSN 0190-9622

Balato A, Balato N, Di Costanzo L, Ayala F (2011). Contact sensitization in the elderly. *Clin Dermatol,* 2011 Vol.29, No.1 (January-February 2011), pp. 24-30, ISSN 0738-081X.

Barros M A, Baptista A, Correia T M, Azevedo F (1991). Patch testing in children: a study of 562 schoolchildren. *Contact Dermatitis,* Vol.25, No.3 (September 1991), pp. 156–159, ISSN 0105-1873

Bo K, Thoresen M, Dalgard F (2008). Smokers report more psoriasis, but not atopic dermatitis or hand eczema: results from a Norwegian population survey among adults. *Dermatology,* Vol.216, No.1 (January 2008), pp. 40-45, ISSN 1018-8665.

Brisman J, Meding B, Jarvholm B (1998). Occurrence of self reported hand eczema in Swedish bakers. *Occup Environ Med,* Vol.55, No.11 (November 1998), pp. 750–754.

Bruckner AL, Weston WL, Morelli JG (2000). Does sensitization to contact allergens begin in infancy? *Pediatrics,* Vol.105, No.1 (january 2000), pp. e3, ISSN 0031-4005

Bruynzeel DP, Diepgen TL, Andersen KE, Brandão FM, Bruze M, Frosch PJ, et al G (2005) Monitoring the European Standard series in 10 centres: 1996-2000. *Contact Dermatitis,* Vol.53, No.3 (September 2005), pp. 146–149, ISSN 0105-1873

Bryld L E, Hindsberger C, Kyvik K O, Agner T, Menné T (2003). Risk factors influencing the development of hand eczema in a population-based twin sample. *Br J* Dermatol, Vol.149, No.6 (December 2003), pp. 1214–1220, ISBN 0007-0963

Carlsen BC, Thyssen JP, Menné T, Meldgaard M, Linneberg A, Nielsen NH, et al (2011). Association between filaggrin null mutations and concomitant atopic dermatitis and contact allergy. *Clin Exp Dermatol,* Vol.36, No.5 (July 2011), pp. 467-472, ISSN 0307-6938.

Cherry N, Meyer JN, Adisesh A, Brooke R, Owen-Smith V, Swales C, Beck MH (2000). Surveillance of occupational skin disease: EPIDERM and OPRA. *Br J Dermatol,* Vol.142, No.6 (June 2000), pp. 1128–1134, ISBN 0007-0963

Coenraads PJ, Goncalo M. Skin diseases with high public health impact. Contact dermatitis (2007). *Eur J Dermatol,* Vol.17, No.6 (November-December 2007), pp. 564-565, ISSN 1167-1122.

Davis JA, Visscher MO, Wickett RR, Hoath SB (2010). Influence of tumour necrosis factor-α polymorphism-308 and atopy on irritant contact dermatitis in healthcare workers. *Contact Dermatitis,* Vol.63, No.6 (December 2010), pp. 320-332, ISSN 0105-1873

de Jongh CM, Khrenova L, Verberk MM, Calkoen F, van Dijk FJ, Voss H, et al (2008). Loss-of-function polymorphisms in the filaggrin gene are associated with an increased susceptibility to chronic irritant contact dermatitis: a case-control study. *Br J Dermatol,* Vol.159, No.3 (September 2008), pp. 621-627, ISBN 0007-0963

Devos SA & Van Der Valk PG. (2002) Epicutaneous patch testing. *Eur J Dermatol,* Vol.12, No.5 (September-October 2002), pp. 506-13, ISSN 1167-1122.

Dickel H, Bruckner T, Berhard-Klimt C, Koch T, Scheidt R, Diepgen TL (2002). Surveillance scheme for occupational skin disease in the Saarland, FRG: first report from BKH-S. *Contact Dermatitis,* Vol.46, No4 (April 2002), pp. 197-206, ISSN 0105-1873

Diepgen TL & Coenrads PJ (2000). The epidemiology of occupational contact dermatitis. In: Kanerva L, Elsner P, Wahlberg JE, Maibach HI (ed). Handbook of occupational dermatology, 1st ed; Springer Verlag berlin Heidelberg New York, ISBN 3-540-064046-0. pp 3-16.

Diepgen TL, Coenraads PJ (2000). The impact of sensitivity, specificity and positive predictive value of patch testing: the more you test, the more you get? *Contact Dermatitis,* Vol.42, No.6 (June 2000), pp. 315-7, ISSN 0105-1873

Dotterud LK, Falk E S (1994). Metal allergy in north Norwegian schoolchildren and its relationship with ear piercing and atopy. *Contact Dermatitis,* Vol.31, No.5 (November 1994), pp. 308–313, ISSN 0105-1873

Dotterud LK, Falk E S (1995). Contact allergy in relation to hand eczema and atopic diseases in north Norwegian schoolchildren. *Acta Paediatr,* Vol.84, No.4 (April 1995), pp. 402–406, ISSN 0001-656X.

Dotterud LK, Smith-Sivertsen T (2007). Allergic contact sensitization in the general adult population: a population-based study from northern Norway. *Contact Dermatitis,* Vol.56, No.1 (January 2007), pp. 10–15, ISSN 0105-1873

Fernández Vozmediano JM, Armario Hita JC (2005). Allergic contact dermatitis in children. *J Eur Acad Dermatol Venereol,* Vol.19, No.1 (January 2005), pp. 42–46, ISSN 0926-9959.

Fowler J F, Duh M S, Chang J, Person J, Thorn D, Raut M, et al (2006). A survey-based assessment of the prevalence and severity of chronic hand dermatitis in a managed care organization. *Cutis,* Vol.77, No.6 (June 2006), pp. 385–392, ISSN 0011-4162.

García-Gavín J, Armario-Hita JC, Fernández-Redondo V, Fernández-Vozmediano JM, Sánchez-Pérez J, Silvestre JF, et al (2011). Epidemiology of Contact Dermatitis in Spain. Results of the Spanish Surveillance System on Contact Allergies for the year 2008. *Actas Dermosifiliogr, Vol.102, No.2 (March 2011), pp.* 98-105, ISSN 0001-7310

Geier J, Struppek K (1995). Amamnese-Auxilium für die berufsdermatologische Untersuchung von Mauren, Betobbauern, Fliesenlegern and Angehörigen verwandter Berufe. *Dermatosen in Beruf und Umwelt,* Vol.43, No.2 (January 1995), pp. 75-80, ISSN 03432432.

Hald M, Berg N D, Elberling J, Johansen J D (2008). Medical consultations in relation to severity of hand eczema in the general population. *Br J Dermatol,* Vol.158, No.4 (April 2008), pp. 773–777, ISSN 0007-0963

Halkier-Sorensen L (1996). Occupational skin diseases. *Contact Dermatitis,* Vol.35, Suppl 1:1-120, ISSN 0105-1873

Hammonds LM, Hall VC, Yiannias JA (2009). Allergic contact dermatitis in 136 children patch tested betweeen 2000 and 2006. *Intern J Dermatol,* Vol.48, No.3 (March 2009), pp. 271-274, ISSN 0011-9059.

Itschner L, Hinnen U, Elsner P (1996) Skin risk assessment of metalworking fluids: A survey among Swiss suppliers. *Dermatology,* Vol.193, No.1 (January 1996), pp. 33-35, ISSN 1421-9832.

Josefson A, Farm G, Stymne B, Meding B (2006). Nickel allergy and hand eczema-a 20-year follow up. *Contact Dermatitis,* Vol.55, No.5 (November 2006), pp. 286–290, ISSN 0105-1873

Kavli G, Forde O H (1984). Hand dermatoses in Tromso. *Contact Dermatitis,* Vol.10, No.3 (March 1984), pp. 174–177, ISSN 0105-1873

Katsarou A, Armenaka M (2011). Atopic dermatitis in older patients: particular points. J Eur Acad Dermatol Venereol, Vol.25, No.1 (January 2011), pp. 12-18, ISSN 0926-9959.

Lammintausta K, Kalimo KM, Fagerlund VL. Patch test reactions in atopic patients. Contact Dermatitis, Vol.26, No.4 (April 1992), pp. 234-240, ISSN 0105-1873.

Lantinga H, Nater J P, Coenraads P J (1984). Prevalence, incidence and course of eczema on the hands and forearms in a sample of the general population. *Contact Dermatitis,* Vol.10, No.3 (March 1984), pp. 135–139, ISSN 0105-1873

Lazarov A (2006). European Standard Series patch test results from a contact dermatitis clinic in Israel during the 7-year period from 1998 to 2004. *Contact Dermatitis,* Vol.55, No.2 (August 2006), pp. 73-76, ISSN 0105-1873

Lerbaek A, Kyvik K O, Ravn H, Menn´e T, Agner T (2007). Incidence of hand eczema in a population-based twin cohort: genetic and environmental risk factors. *Br J Dermatol,* Vol.157, No.3 (September 2007), pp. 552–557, ISSN 0007-0963

Lewis VJ, Statham BN, Chowdhury MMU (2004). Allergic contact dermatitis in 191 consecutively patch tested children. *Contact Dermatitis,* Vol.51, No.3 (September 2004), pp. 155–156, ISSN 0105-1873

Lind M L, Albin M, Brisman J, Kronholm Diab K, Lillienberg L, Mikoczy Z, et al (2007) Incidence of hand eczema in female Swedish hairdressers. *Occup Environ Med,* Vol.64, No.3 (March 2007), pp. 191-195, ISSN 1351-0711.

McCurdy SA, Wiggins TH, Seligman PJ, Halperin WE (1990). Assessing dermatitis in epidemiologic studies: occupational skin disease among California grape and tomato harvesters. *Am J Ind Med,* Vol.16, No.2 (March-April 1990), pp. 147-157, ISSN 0271-3586

McFadden JP, Dearman RJ, White JM, Basketter DA, Kimber I (2011). The Hapten-Atopy hypothesis II: the 'cutaneous hapten paradox'. *Clin Exp Allergy,* Vol.41, No.3 (March 2011), pp. 327-337, ISSN 0954-7894

Meding B (1990). Epidemiology of hand eczema in an industrial city. *Acta Derm Venereol Suppl (Stockh),* Vol.153, No.1 (January 1990), pp. 1–43, ISSN 0365-8341.

Meding B, Lidén C, Berglind N (2001). Self-diagnosed dermatitis in adults. Results from a population survey in Stockholm. *Contact Dermatitis,* Vol.45, No.6 (December 2001); pp. 341–345, ISSN 0105-1873

Meding B, Jarvholm B (2002). Hand eczema in Swedish adults – changes in prevalence between 1983 and 1996. *J Invest Dermatol,* Vol.118, No.4 (April 2002), pp. 719–723, ISSN 0022-202X

Meding B, Jarvholm B (2004). Incidence of hand eczema-a population-based retrospective study. *J Invest Dermatol,* Vol.122, No.4 (April 2004), pp. 873–877, ISSN 0022-202X

Meding B, Swanbeck G (1987). Prevalence of hand eczema in an industrial city. *Br J Dermatol,* Vol.116, No.5 (May 1987), pp. 627–634, ISSN 0007-0963

Meding B, Swanbeck G. Predictive factors for hand eczema (1990). *Contact Dermatitis,* Vol.23, No.3 (September 1990), pp. 154–161, ISSN 0105-1873

Meding B, Wrangsjö K, Hosseiny S, Andersson E, Hagberg S, Toren K, et al (2006). Occupational skin exposure and hand eczema among dental technicians-need for improved prevention. *Scand J Work Environ Health,* Vol.32, No.3 (June 2006), pp. 219–224, ISSN 0355-3140

Meijer C, Bredberg M, Fischer T, Widstrom L (1995). Ear piercing, and nickel and cobalt sensitization, in 520 young Swedish men doing compulsory military service. *Contact Dermatitis,* Vol.32, No.3 (March 1995), pp. 147–149, ISSN 0105-1873

Meneghini CL, Angelini G (1984). Primary and secondary sites of occupational contact dermatitis. *Dermatosen in Beruf und Umwelt,* Vol.32, No.6 (November-December 1984), pp. 205-207, ISSN 03432432.

Menné T, Borgan O, Green A (1982). Nickel allergy and hand dermatitis in a stratified sample of the Danish female population: an epidemiological study including a statistic appendix. *Acta Derm Venereol,* Vol.62, No.1 (January 1982), pp. 35–41, ISSN 0001-5555

Menné T, Knudsen B (1997). Clinical data in the classification of contact allergens. In: Flyvholm A-A-, Andersen KE, baranski B, Sarlo K (eds). Criteria for classification of skin and airway-sensitizing substances in the work and general environments. *WHO Regional Office for Europ*e, Copenhagen, pp 91-100, EUR/ICP/EHPM 05 02 01.

Moberg C, Alderling M, Meding B (2009). Hand eczema and quality of life: a population-based study. Br *J Dermatol,* Vol.161, No.2 (August 2009), pp. 397-403, ISSN 0007-0963

Modjtahedi SP, Maibach HI. Ethnicity as a possible endogenous factor in irritant contact dermatitis: comparing the irritant response among Caucasians, blacks, and Asians (2002). Contact Dermatitis, Vol.47, No.5 (November 2002), pp. 272-278, ISSN 0105-1873

Montnemery P, Nihlen U, Lofdahl C G, Nyberg P, Svensson A (2005). Prevalence of hand eczema in an adult Swedish population and the relationship to risk occupation and smoking. *Acta Derm Venereol,* Vol.85, No.5 (September 2005), pp. 429–432, ISSN 0001-5555

Mortz CG, Lauritsen JM, Bindslev-Jensen C, Andersen KE (2001). Prevalence of atopic dermatitis, asthma, allergic rhinitis, and hand and contact dermatitis in adolescents. The Odense Adolescence Cohort Study on Atopic Diseases and Dermatitis. *Br J Dermatol,* Vol.144, No.3 (March 2001), pp. 523-532, ISSN 0007-0963

Mortz C G, Lauritsen J M, Bindslev-Jensen C, Andersen K E (2002). Contact allergy and allergic contact dermatitis in adolescents: prevalence measures and associations. The Odense Adolescence Cohort Study on Atopic Diseases and Dermatitis (TOACS). *Acta Derm Venereol,* Vol.82, No.5 (September 2002), pp. 352–358, ISSN 0001-5555

Muñoz Lejarazu D (2009). Contact dermatitis: Alergológica-2005. *J Investig Allergol Clin Immunol, Vol.19,* Suppl 2:34-6, ISSN 1018-9068

Nedorost ST, Stevens SR. Diagnosis and treatment of allergic skin disorders in the elderly. Drugs. *Drugs Aging,* 2001 Vol.18, No.11 (December 2001), pp. 827-835, ISSN 1170-229X.

Nielsen NH, Linneberg A, Menné T, Madsen F, Frolund L, Dirksen A, et al (2001a) Allergic contact sensitization in an adult Danish population: two cross-sectional surveys eight years apart (the Copenhagen Allergy Study). *Acta Derm Venereol,* Vol.81, No.1 (January-February 2001), pp. 31-4, ISSN 0001-5555

Nielsen NH, Linneberg A, Menné T, Madsen F, Frolund L, Dirksen A, et al (2001b). Persistence of contact allergy among Danish adults: an 8-year follow-up study. *Contact Dermatitis,* Vol.45, No.6 (December 2001), pp. 350-353, ISSN 0105-1873

Nielsen N H, Linneberg A, Menne T, Madsen F, Frølund L, Dirksen A, Jørgensen T (2002a). The association between contact allergy and hand eczema in 2 cross-sectional surveys 8 years apart. *Contact Dermatitis,* Vol.47, No.2 (August 2002), pp. 71–77, ISSN 0105-1873

Nielsen N H, Linneberg A, Menné T, Madsen F, Frølund L, Dirksen A, et al (2002b). Incidence of allergic contact sensitization in Danish adults between 1990 and 1998; the Copenhagen Allergy Study, Denmark. *Br J Dermatol,* Vol.147, No.3 (September 2002), pp. 487–492, ISSN 0007-0963

Nielsen N H, Menne T (1992). Allergic contact sensitization in an unselected Danish population. The Glostrup Allergy Study, Denmark. *Acta Derm Venereol,* Vol.72, No.6 (November 1992), pp. 456–460, ISSN 0001-5555

Ortengren U, Andreasson H, Karlsson S, Meding B, Barregard L (1999). Prevalence of self-reported hand eczema and skin symptoms associated with dental materials among Swedish dentists. *Eur J Oral Sci,* Vol.107, No.6 (December 1999), pp. 496–505, ISSN 0909-8836

Peltonen L (1979). Nickel sensitivity in the general population. *Contact Dermatitis,* Vol.5, No.1 (January 1979), pp. 27–32, ISSN 0105-1873

Prakash AV, Davis MD (2010) Contact dermatitis in older adults: a review of the literature. *Am J Clin Dermatol,* 2010 Vol.11, No.6 (December 2010), pp. 373-381, ISSN: 1175-0561.

Robinson MK. Population differences in skin structure and physiology and the susceptibility to irritant and allergic contact dermatitis: implications for skin safety testing and risk assessment (1999). *Contact Dermatitis,* Vol.41, No.2 (August 1999), pp. 65-79, ISSN 0105-1873

Rockl H, Muller E, Hiltermann W (1966). On the prognostic value of positive skin tests in infants and children. *Arch Klin Exp Dermatol,* Vol.226, No.4 (October 1966), pp. 407–419, ISSN 0300-8614

Ruff CA, Belsito DV (2006). The impact of various patient factors on contact allergy to nickel, cobalt, and chromate. *J Am Acad Dermatol,* Vol.55, No.1 (July 1966), pp. 32-39, ISSN 0190-9622

Rui F, Bovenzi M, Prodi A, Fortina AB, Romano I, Peserico A, et al (2010). Nickel, cobalt and chromate sensitization and occupation. *Contact Dermatitis,* Vol.62, No.4 (April 2010), pp. 225-231, ISSN 0105-1873

Saint-Mezard P, Rosieres A, Krasteva M, Berard F, Dubois B, Kaiserlian D et al. Allergic contact dermatitis (2004). *Eur J Dermatol,* Vol.14, No.5 (September-October 2004), pp. 284-295, ISSN 1167-1122

Schafer T, Bohler E, Ruhdorfer S, Weigl L, Wessner D, Filipiak B, et al (2001). Epidemiology of contact allergy in adults. *Allergy,* Vol.56, No.12 (December 2001), pp. 1192–1196, ISSN 0105-4538

Schnuch A, Uter W, Geier J, Frosch PJ, Rustemeyer TH (1998). Contact allergies in health care workers. *Acta derm Venereol Stockh,* Vol.78, No.5 (September 1998), pp. 358-363, ISSN 0365-8341.

Seidenari S, Giusti F, Pepe P, Mantovani L (2005). Contact sensitization in 1094 children undergoing patch testing over a 7-year period. *Pediatr Dermatol,* Vol.22, No.1 (January-February 2005), pp. 1–5, On-line ISSN 1525-1470.

Smit HA, Van Rijssen A, Vandenbroucke J, Coenraads PJ. (1994) Susceptibility to and incidence of hand dermatitis in a cohort of apprentice hairdressers and nurses. *Scand J Work Environ Health,* Vol.20, No.2 (April 1994), pp. 113-121, ISSN 0355-3140

Sosted H, Hesse U, Menne T, Andersen KE, Johansen JD (2005). Contact dermatitis to hair dyes in a Danish adult population: an interview-based study. *Br J Dermatol,* Vol.153, No.1 (july 2005), pp. 132-135, ISSN 0007-0963

Svedman C, Ekqvist S, Möller H, Bjork J, Gruvberger B, Holmstrom E, Bruze M (2007). Unexpected sensitization routes and general frequency of contact allergies in an elderly stented Swedish population. *Contact Dermatitis,* Vol.56, No.6 (June 2007), pp. 338–343, ISSN 0105-1873

Thyssen JP, Linneberg A, Menné T, Johansen JD (2007). The epidemiology of contact allergy in the general population - prevalence and main findings. *Contact Dermatitis, Vol.57, No.5 (November 2007); pp.* 287-99, ISSN 0105-1873

Thyssen JP, Linneberg A, Menne T, Nielsen NH, Johansen JD (2009). The prevalence and morbidity of sensitization to fragrance mix I in the general population. *Br J Dermatol,* Vol.161, No.1 (July 2009), pp. 95-101, ISSN 0007-0963

Thyssen JP, Johansen JD, Linneberg A, Menné T (2010). The epidemiology of hand eczema in the general population - prevalence and main findings. *Contact Dermatitis, Vol.62, No.2 (February 2010), pp.* 75-87, ISSN 0105-1873

Thyssen JP, Johansen JD, Menné T, Nielsen NH, Linneberg A (2010). Effect of tobacco smoking and alcohol consumption on the prevalence of nickel sensitization and contact sensitization. *Acta Derm Venereol,* Vol.90, No.1 (January 2010), pp. 27-33, ISSN 0001-5555

Uter W, Rämsch C, Aberer W, Ayala F, Balato A, Beliauskiene A, et al (2009). The European baseline series in 10 European Countries, 2005/2006 - results of the European Surveillance System on Contact Allergies (ESSCA). *Contact Dermatitis,* Vol.61, No.1 (July 2009), pp. 31-38, ISSN 0105-1873

Uveges RE, Grimwood RE, Slawsky LD, Marks JG Jr (1995) Epidemiology of hand dermatitis in dental personnel. *Mil* Med, Vol.160, No.7 (July 1995), pp. 335-338, ISSN 0026-4075

Weston W L, Weston J A, Kinoshita J, Kloepfer S, Carreon L, Toth S, Bullard D, Harper K, Martinez S (1986). Prevalence of positive epicutaneous tests among infants, children, and adolescents. *Pediatrics,* Vol.78, No.6 (December 1986), pp. 1070–1074, ISSN 0031-4005

Yngveson M, Svensson A, Johannisson A, Isacsson A (2000). Hand dermatosis in upper secondary school pupils: 2-year comparison and follow-up. *Br J Dermatol,* Vol.142, No.3 (March 2000), pp. 485–489, ISSN 0007-0963

Part 2

Pathogenesis

2

Animal Models of Contact Dermatitis

Federico Simonetta and Christine Bourgeois
INSERM U1012, Université Paris-SUD, UMR-S1012, Le Kremlin-Bicêtre
France

1. Introduction

Contact dermatitis is an inflammatory disease of the skin resulting from direct contact with foreign substances. Understanding the immunological processes that cause the disease is therefore essential for the development of new therapeutic strategies.

Murine models of chemically induced dermatitis have played an essential role in our understanding of the pathophysiology of contact dermatitis, unraveling the role played by inflammatory mediators and identifying potential targets for therapeutic interventions.

In the present chapter we review data obtained in animal models of allergic and irritant contact dermatitis and provide basic protocols to reliably induce contact dermatitis.

A major intent of this chapter is to highlight the respective role of innate and adaptive immune cells in contact dermatitis pathogenesis as revealed by murine studies. Through genetic ablation of single molecules or depletion of specific cell subsets, murine studies provide novel insight on the role of different components of the immune system in the development of contact dermatitis. We review the experimental evidence revealing the role of different T cell subsets in contact dermatitis development, focusing our attention on mechanisms responsible for maintenance or disruption of immune-tolerance. Our analyses will focus on molecular pathways which are promising candidates as targets of future biological therapies.

2. Allergic contact dermatitis

Most of our knowledge on the pathophysiology of contact dermatitis is derived from murine models of Allergic Contact Dermatitis (ACD), a T cell mediated delayed-type hypersensitivity reaction also referred to as contact hypersensitivity (CHS). In this model, skin inflammation is induced by topical application on the epidermis of sensitizing chemical agents which act as haptens (Eisen et al., 1952).

Haptens can be defined as low molecular weight chemicals which are not immunogenic by themselves and that generate new antigenic determinants by binding to epidermal proteins. The reactive haptens commonly employed for ACD induction in murine models include oxazolone (OX), dinitrochlorobenzene (DNCB), dinitrofluorobenzene (DNFB), trinitrochlorobenzene (TNCB), picryl chloride (PI), and fluorescein isothiocyanate (FITC).

Such widely employed haptens are all strong contact allergens exhibiting high proinflammatory capacities which therefore differ from the vast majority of chemicals responsible for human ACD. Importantly recent studies have reproduced the conclusions drawn with strong allergens by using weak haptens (Vocanson et al., 2006; Vocanson et al., 2009) which are more close to those encountered in clinical practice.

2.1 Phases of ACD

Three temporally distinct phases can be identified in ACD: the **sensitization phase**, the **elicitation phase** and the **resolution phase**.

The **sensitization phase,** also referred to as the afferent phase or induction phase, occurs at the first skin contact with a hapten (Fig. 1A). This phase lasts 10–15 days in humans and 5-7 days in mice. Most of employed haptens induce local inflammation by acting on innate immunity receptors (see section 4.1). Activation of the skin innate immunity induces the production of mediators (IL-18, IL-1β, TNF-α, ATP, PGE2, LTB4, ROS, histamine, CCL20) by resident skin cells. These mediators are able to induce the recruitment, migration and activation of cutaneous antigen presenting cells (APC). The skin contains a dense network of APC constituted by two phenotypically and spatially distinct subsets: Langerhans cells (LC), which are located in the epidermal layer of the skin, and dermal DCs (dDC). In addition to skin resident APC, circulating CCR2+ monocytes are rapidly recruited from blood to skin and locally differentiate into dendritic cells. Once activated, APC phagocyte haptenated proteins and migrate from the skin to the para-cortical area of draining lymph nodes (Kripke et al., 1990). There, APC present haptenated peptides through MHC classes I and II molecules at their cell surface (Weltzien et al., 1996) to hapten-specific CD8+ and CD4+ T lymphocytes thus inducing their priming and expansion (Bour et al., 1995 ; Xu H et al., 1996 ; Krasteva et al., 1998). Primed hapten-specific T cells can then emigrate from the lymph nodes and enter the blood from which they recirculate to different tissues including the skin.

The **elicitation phase**, also referred to as the efferent or challenge phase, occurs after subsequent challenges with the same hapten to which a host has been previously sensitized (Fig. 1B). This efferent phase of CHS takes place within 72 hours upon exposure to the allergen in humans and 24 to 48 hours in mice. Once more, haptenated peptides are uptaken by skin APC which present to hapten specific primed T cells patrolling in the skin. As this process directly takes place on the site of inflammation and as T cells activated at this stage are already primed cells, the elicitation phase develops extremely rapidly.

Activated T cells produce effector cytokines, notably IFN-γ and IL-17 (see section 4.2), which activate skin resident cells which in turn secrete cytokines and chemokines pertaining cell recruitment at exposure site. Continuous recruitment of circulating cells then leads to polymorphous cellular infiltrate and persistence of the inflammatory reaction over several days.

The **resolution phase**, during which the inflammatory response progressively disappears, then follows. This phase presumably results from down-regulating mechanisms including passive processes, such as the progressive disappearance of the hapten from the epidermis, as well as active cellular processes, such as the intervention of regulatory T cells (see section 5).

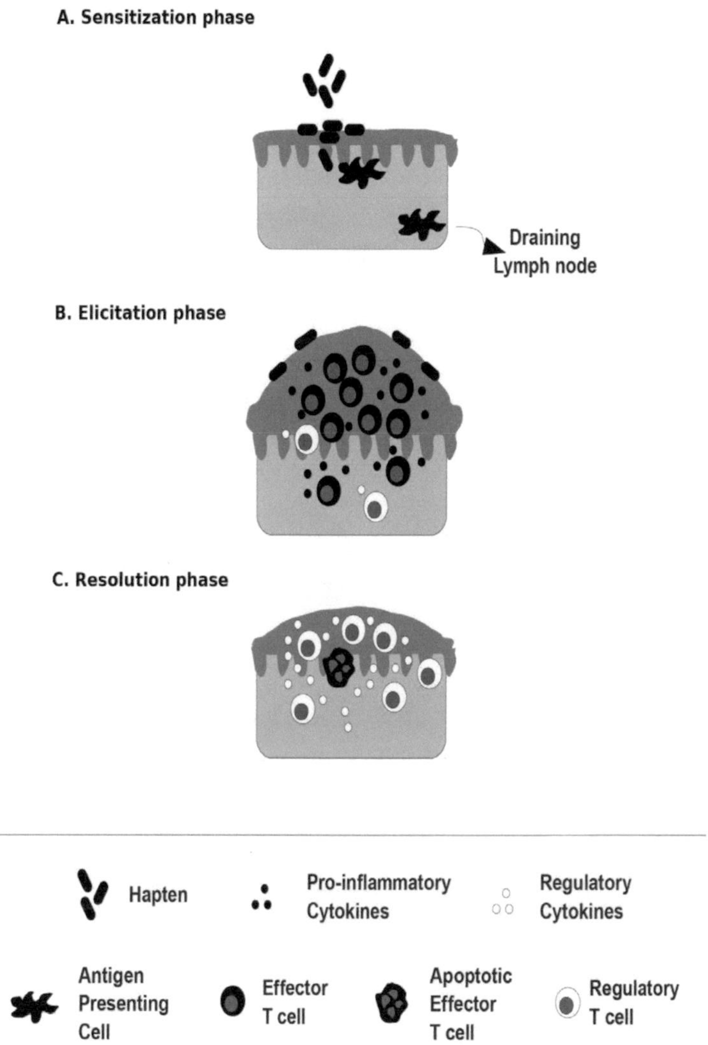

Fig. 1. Schematic representation of the pathophysiology of the different phases of allergic contact dermatitis. (A) the sensitization phase (B) the elicitation phase (C) the resolution phase.

2.2 Experimental protocol

Experimental protocol for ACD induction is graphically summarized in Figure 2. For sensitization, mice are painted at day 0 on the shaved back (or abdomen) with 100 µl of DNFB 0.5% in a 4:1 mixture of acetone and olive oil. Mice are challenged 6 days later by application of 20 µl DNFB 0.2% in olive oil (10 µl to each side of one ear). Ear thickness is measured with a digital calliper before challenge and at 24-48 hours after treatment. Ear swelling is calculated by subtracting the value recorded for vehicle-control ear from the hapten-applied ear. Histological examination can be performed in order to confirm changes in ear thickness and to quantify cellular infiltration. Moreover, lymphocytes infiltrating inflamed skin can be investigated by FACS analysis after isolation. In figure 4 we provide a detailed protocol to isolate lymphocytes from skin.

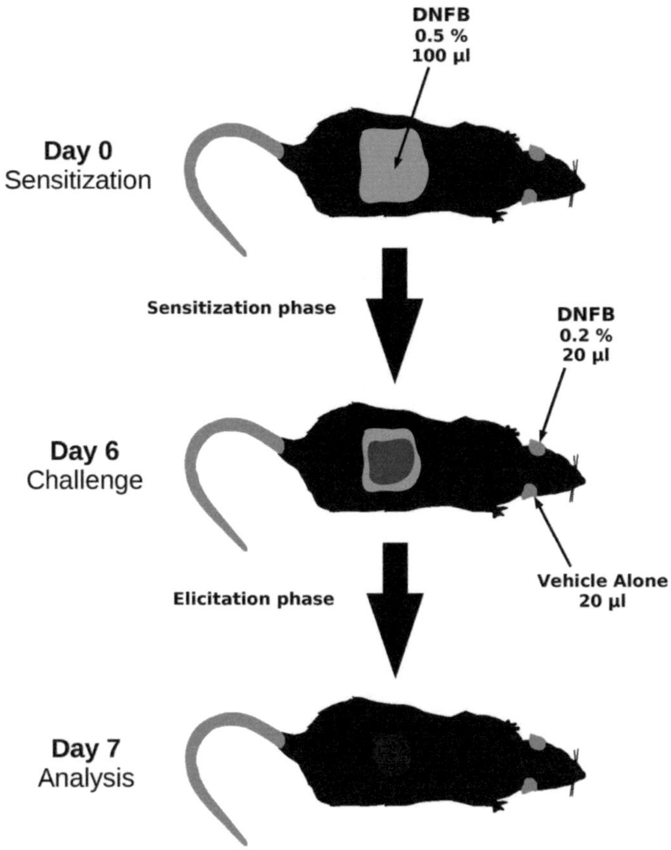

Fig. 2. Allergic contact dermatitis experimental protocol.

3. Irritant contact dermatitis

Clinical evidence indicates that a primary, irritative form of contact dermatitis can develop upon a single first contact with chemicals in previously unsensitized patients.

Irritant contact dermatitis (ICD), also known as "primary ACD" or "primary CHS" develops upon skin exposure to strong haptens such as urushiol, primine, DNFB and DNCB (Kanerva et al., 1994).

ICD is the result of the liberation of proinflammatory mediators upon skin exposed to haptens which in turn promote recruitment from blood of inflammatory cells to tissue sites. The magnitude of ICD is similar to that of classical ACD but presents a different kinetic since the onset of the skin inflammation is delayed in ICD by 5 days, a time period needed to achieve T cell priming.

The eczematous lesions of ICD are morphologically indistinguishable from those present in conventional ACD, suggesting that common mechanisms could be involved in the two processes. Importantly, using an experimental murine model of primary CHS induced by a single DNFB or FITC painting on mice ears without subsequent challenge, Saint-Mezard and colleagues were able to show that the pathophysiology of one-step ICD is identical to that of two-step classical ACD, involving the same effector and down-regulating immune mechanisms (Saint-Mezard et al., 2003). Remarkably, ICD responses were strictly dose-dependent and reproducibly more important in C57Bl/6 mice than in BALB mice (Bonneville et al., 2007). More importantly, Bonneville et al. demonstrated an inter-relationship between ICD and ACD and showed that upon hapten rechallenge the intensity of ACD reaction is proportional to the magnitude of the former ICD response (Bonneville et al., 2007).

3.1 Experimental protocol

Experimental protocol for ICD induction is graphically summarized in Figure 3. Naive mice are exposed at day 0 to a single application of 20 µl of DNFB 0.5% in a 4:1 mixture of acetone and olive oil applied on the left ear, while the same volume of vehicle alone is applied on the right ear as a control. Six days after ear sensitization, ear thickness is measured with a digital calliper. Analysis can be performed similarly to ACD model (see section 2.1).

4. Effector mechanisms in allergic contact dermatitis

4.1 Role of innate immunity

ACD is a delayed type hypersensitivity reaction. Despite being a prototypical T cell mediated response, a role of innate immunity has been pointed out since early studies and has been recently better elucidated. A common feature of contact allergens employed in experimental studies is their local irritancy and their capacity to act as adjuvants. This feature depends on their ability to activate the innate immune system.

Innate immune system cells express pattern recognition receptors (PRRs), germ-line encoded receptors that recognize so-called pathogen-associated molecular patterns (PAMPs), microbial molecular structures such as bacterial or fungal cell wall components, microbial nucleic acids, proteins or sugars. Depending on their localization we can distinguish transmembrane PRRs, such as Toll-like receptors (TLRs) which recognize PAMPs in the extracellular space and/or in phagosomes or endosomes, and cytosolic PRRs, such as nucleotide-binding oligomerization domain containing (Nod)-like receptors (NLR).

Investigating the involvement of TLRs in the development of CHS to contact allergens, Martin and coworkers first revealed a crucial role for TLR2 and TLR4 (Martin et al., 2008). Mice lacking both TLR4 and TLR2 were resistant to TNCB induced CHS, thus establishing a link between hapten-induced inflammation and innate immune-responses. Accordingly, mice deficient for MyD88, a molecule centrally involved in TLRs signaling trunsduction, failed to mount CHS responses to DNFB (Klekotka et al., 2010). Further evidence for a role of TLRs in cutaneous ACD comes from a study on Nickel (Ni(2+)), by far one of the most relevant contact allergens in terms of incidence of contact eczema and sensitization rates. Schmidt et al., identified human TLR4 as the crucial mediator of the innate immune response to Ni(2+) (Schmidt M et al., 2010). After having provided in vitro evidence for the need of TLR4 expression for Ni(2+) induced activation, the authors demonstrated that transgenic expression of hTLR4 in TLR4-deficient mice confers sensitivity of naturally resistant mice to Ni(2+)-induced CHS. Those results formally demonstrate that Ni(2+) employs TLR4, a signaling component of the antibacterial defense system, to elicit its allergic reactions.

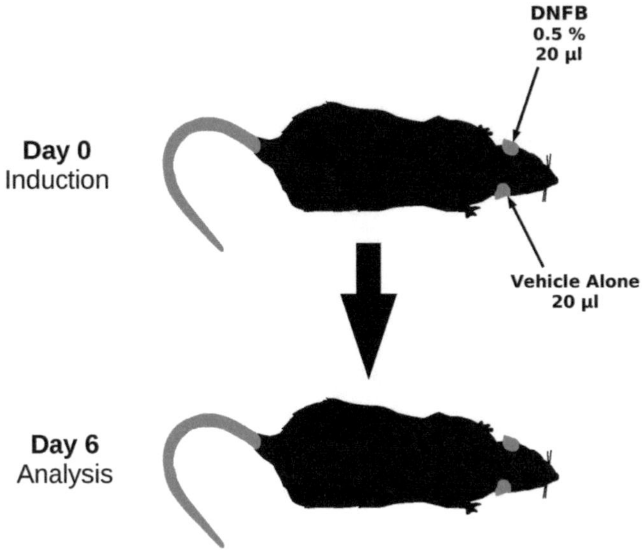

Fig. 3. Irritant contact dermatitis experimental protocol.

NLRP3, also known as NALP3/Cryopyrin/CIAS1/PYPAF1, belongs to the NLR family of PRRs and is activated by a variety of pathogen- and host-derived "danger" signals including: whole pathogens (Candida albicans, Saccharomyces cerevisiae, Staphylococcus aureus, Listeria monocytogenes); pathogen-associated molecules (bacterial pore–forming toxins and malarial hemozoin); environmental irritants (silica, asbestos, ultraviolet light); host-derived "danger-associated molecular patterns" (ATP, glucose, monosodium urate, calcium pyrophosphate dihydrate, amyloid β, hyaluronan); and immune adjuvants (aluminum salt). NLRP3 forms a multi-protein complex, known as the NLRP3 inflammasome, together with the adaptor protein apoptosis-associated specklike protein (ASC) and caspase-1. Inflammasome activation leads to the proteolysis to bioactive form of the proinflammatory cytokines IL-1β and IL-18. Langherans cells and keratinocytes can secrete IL-1β and IL-18 upon exposure to sensitizing agents (Sauder etal., 1984 ; Enk et al., 1993 ; Nail et al., 1999) and these cytokines are crucial for Langherans cells migration to the draining lymph nodes (Cumberbatch et al., 2002). It is therefore not surprising that NLRP3 inflammasome and IL-1/IL-1R signaling are required for ACD development. Shornick and colleagues first demonstrated that IL-1β deficient mice showed defective CHS responses to topically applied TNCB and that this defect could be overcome by local intradermal injection of recombinant IL-1β immediately before antigen application (Shornick et al., 1996). Accordingly, as NLRP3 inflammasome activation is necessary for active IL-1β production, mice lacking either NLRP3, the adaptor protein ASC or caspase-1 showed impaired CHS responses to TNCB and DNFB (Sutterwala et al., 2006 ; Watanabe et al., 2007 ; Antonopoulos et al., 2001). Finally, IL-1R deficiency (Klekotka et al., 2010) or treatment of mice with the IL-1R antagonist (Kondo et al., 1995) efficiently prevented CHS development.

Production of IL-18, a cytokine with structural similarities to IL-1β, is also regulated by NLRP3 inflammasome activation. In vivo studies showed that CHS responses to oxazolone and DNFB were significantly inhibited in mice treated with neutralizing IL-18 Ab (Wang et al., 2002) or which were deficient for either IL-18 (Antonopoulos et al., 2008) or IL-18R (Klekotka et al., 2010). Interestingly CHS could be rescued by local intradermal administration of IL-18 prior to sensitization, in agreement with an implication of IL-18 in the afferent phase of the disease.

Trying to dissect the relative contribution of IL-1β and IL-18 in ACD development, Antonopoulos et al., further showed that IL-1β but not IL-18 administration was able to rescue the defective CHS response observed in caspase-1-/- mice, which have no functional IL-1β or IL-18 (Antonopoulos et al., 2008). Therefore IL-1β appears to be the main caspase-1-dependent inducer of inflammation in CHS.

4.2 Role of adaptive immunity

ACD is a cellular immune reaction which has been identified since early studies as mediated primarily by T cells. Adoptive transfer of T cells from sensitized mice into non-sensitized recipients results in the transfer of sensitization (Moorhead et al., 1978 ; van Loveren et al., 1983). Moreover, T cell depletion before the elicitation phase results in complete abolition of the reaction (Gocinski and Tigelaar, 1990).

As ACD is a classical DTH reaction and since cutaneous infiltrates in humans show a clear preponderance of CD4+ T cells, ACD has first being considered to be mediated primarily by CD4 T cells. However, based on contrasting experimental results, the role exerted by different T cell subsets in the physiopathology of the disease has longly been debated.

In some experimental models CD4 T cells have indeed been shown to mediate the allergic response (Miller and Jenkins, 1985 ; Gocinski and Tigelaar 1990 ; Kohler et al., 1995 ; Wang B et al., 2000). However, most studies agree in identifying CD8+ T cells as the main effector compartment in ACD to different haptens (Gocinski and Tigelaar, 1990 ; Bour et al, 1995 ; Xu et al, 1996 ; Bouloc et al, 1998 ; Kehren et al., 1999 ; Martin et al., 2000 ; Akiba et al., 2002 ; Dubois et al., 2003 ; Saint-Mezard et al., 2004).

Such evidence pointing to a role of CD8 T cells in ACD has been obtained through several experimental approaches such as in vivo depletion of normal mice with anti-CD4 and anti-CD8 mAbs, use of MHC class I-/- CD8+ T cell-deficient mice and MHC class II-/- CD4+ T cell-deficient mice or adoptive transfer of purified primed CD4+ and/or CD8+ T cells from sensitized mice into naïve recipients.

Using the antibody depletion model, Gocinski and Tigelaar showed that CD8 depletion prior to DNFB sensitisation led to a substantial reduction of ear swelling upon rechallenge, for the first time (Gocinski and Tigelaar, 1990) pointing to CD8 T cells as major players in ACD. Even more surprisingly, the authors demonstrated that when CD4 T cells were depleted prior to sensitization with DNFB, rather than observing a reduction in ear swelling upon rechallenge, responses were augmented suggesting that CD4 T cells were indeed behaving as down-regulatory cells. These conclusions were subsequently confirmed by Bour et al. studying CHS in MHC class I and MHC class II knockout mice, which are deficient in CD8+ and CD4+ T cells, respectively. In this system, Class I deficient mice failed to develop DNFB-induced CHS responses while class II deficient mice developed an enhanced CHS reaction (Bour et al., 1995).

An explanation to these phenomena came from the demonstration that upon sensitization with DNFB or oxaloxone hapten-loaded APC migrated to draining lymph nodes from the skin induce the differentiation of IFN-γ-producing effector CD8+ T cells and IL-4/IL-10-producing CD4+ T cells that negatively regulate the response (Xu et al., 1996). Since CD8+ effector T cells primarily exert their function through cytotoxicity, the demonstration of a central role of CD8 T cells in CHS leads to investigate whether cytotoxicity mediated skin inflammation. Kehren et al. showed that mice double deficient in perforin and FasL were able to develop hapten-specific CD8+ T cells in the lymphoid organs but did not show CHS reaction in the skin, thus demonstrating that the CHS reaction is dependent on CD8+ T cells cytotoxic activity (Kehren et al., 1999). Using immunohistochemistry and RT-PCR analysis Akiba and colleagues extended those results by demonstrating that epidermal keratinocytes were the target cells of hapten-specific CD8+ T cells cytotoxicity (Akiba et al., 2002).

Tissue Preparation	**1 -** Sacrifice mice **2 -** Isolate ears **3 -** Separate the two sheets of ear skin with forceps **4 -** Finely cut the tissue with scissors
Tissue Digestion	**5 -** Incubate tissue fragments in Liberase (Roche) 400 µg/ml freshly diluted in PBS for 1 hour at 37°C while shaking
Cells Isolation	**6 -** Vortex vigorously for 1 min **7 -** Pass the suspension through a 70-µm cell strainer **8 -** Press digested tissue through the cell strainer **9 -** Add PBS **10 -** Centrifuge 10 min at 1800 rpm **11 -** Carefully remove the supernatant **12 -** Repeat steps 9-11 **13 -** Resuspend in a 35% Percoll solution (Sigma-Aldrich) **14 -** Centrifuge 25 min at 2500 without brake **15 -** Carefully discard supernatant **16 -** Resuspend the cell pellet in PBS **17 -** Wash twice

Fig. 4. Skin infiltrating lymphocytes preparation for FACS analysis

In addition to the aforementioned role of perforin and FasL, IFN-γ has been shown to play an important role in CHS responses and a defect in IFN-γ signals as a result of the genetic disruption of the IFN-γR2 gene (Lu et al., 1998) or of the IFN-γ encoding gene (Wakabayashi et al., 2005) suppresses CHS responses. However other reports failed to confirm impaired CHS responses in mice with IFN-γ signaling disruption (Saulnier et al., 1995 ; Reeve et al., 1999). Moreover, neutralization of IFN-γ in DNFB sensitized mice before challenge failed to suppress the elicitation of CHS (He et al., 2006).

Searching for other mediatiors of CHS, Nakae et al. reported that CHS was reduced in IL-17 knockout mice compared with wild-type controls (Nakae et al., 2002). Subsequently, IL-17 neutralization in DNFB sensitized mice before challenge has been shown to suppress the elicitation of CHS (He et al., 2006). IL-17 is a well known chemotactic factor and absence of IL-17 signaling inhibited the infiltration of T cells, monocytes/macrophages and granulocytes into hapten-challenged skin tissues. Interestingly, He and coworkers demonstrated that in the DNFB induced CHS model CD8+ T cells represents the major source of IL-17 at the inflammation site. Moreover, CD8+ IL-17-producing T cell subpopulation is distinct from CD8+ IFN-γ-producing T cells and is important in effector functions during the elicitation of CHS. Subsequently the same group extended those results and demonstrated that IL-17 and IFN-γ signaling are both required for optimal elicitation of CHS by probably acting through distinguished mechanisms (He et al., 2009).

Globally, murine studies allowed to identify CD8+ T cells as the major cellular player in ACD pathogenesis and pointed out several molecular pathways which can be taken into account for the development of immuno-therapeutic strategies.

5. Regulatory mechanisms in allergic contact dermatitis

Both sensitization to chemicals and the effector phase of contact allergy are highly regulated events. This task is guaranteed by multiple mechanisms, including antigen-presenting cells and effector T cells apoptosis, production and release of anti-inflammatory mediators and action of a specialized subset of T lymphocytes with down-regulatory properties known as regulatory T cells.

Regulatory T cells (Treg) are a critical CD4 T cell subset involved in the control of immune homeostasis and in regulation of inflammation (Sakaguchi et al., 2008). Treg represent about 5-10% of the whole T cell compartment and are characterized by the preferential expression of several molecules including CD25, the alpha chain of IL-2 receptor (Sakaguchi et al., 1995), and FOXP3, a transcription factor which is necessary for Treg development and function (Fontenot et al., 2003).

CD4+CD25+ Treg cells have been implicated in the control CHS responses to haptens in mice. The first evidence of such a role for Treg cells came from a study investigating the mechanisms responsible for the "oral tolerance" phenomenon (Dubois et al., 2003). It was known that DNFB oral administration prior to sensibilisation could induce a tolerant state and prevent the development of ACD (Garside et al., 2001). Desvignes and coworkers showed that tolerance induction was dependent on the presence of CD4 T cells (Desvignes et al., 1996 ; Desvignes et al., 2000) suggesting the implication of a CD4 T cell subset with regulatory characteristics. Using in vivo models of adoptive transfer and antibody depletion of CD4+CD25+ cells, Dubois et al. demonstrated that naturally occurring CD4+CD25+ T cells are instrumental for orally induced tolerance and control hapten-specific CD8+ T cell responses mediating skin inflammation (Dubois et al., 2003).

Further studies confirmed the role of Treg cells in classical ACD reaction. Depletion of CD4+ CD25+ T cells by in vivo treatment of mice with an anti-CD25 mAb at the time of sensitization led to an increased CD8+ T cell priming and an enhanced ACD reaction (Kish et al., 2005). Conversely, IL-2-IgG2b fusion protein treatment of mice induces a decreased ACD reaction associated with an increase in the CD4+ CD25+ Treg cell numbers (Ruckert et al., 2002).

Importantly, a role for CD4+ CD25+ Treg cells in maintaining immune tolerance to skin allergens has been confirmed in humans. Cavani et al. showed that CD4+ T cells isolated from the peripheral blood of six healthy nonallergic individuals showed a limited capacity to proliferate in response to nickel in vitro, but responsiveness was strongly augmented by CD25+ Treg depletion (Cavani et al. 2003).

Mechanisms involved in Treg maintenance of skin tolerance still remain to be fully elucidated. As IL-10 has been shown to mediate in vivo Treg suppression in other murine models of disease, it has been evaluated in the context of ACD. IL-10 has been shown to participate in restoring oral tolerance to haptens induced by CD4+ T cells (Dubois et al., 2003). Subsequently Ring et al. showed that Treg cells injection into sensitized mice at the time of local hapten challenge significantly inhibited influx of effector T cells into inflamed skin tissue, but that this effect was abrogated when CD4+CD25+ Treg cells isolated from IL-10–/– mice were transferred (Ring et al., 2006). More recently, Rudensky and coworkers generated mice in which Treg cell-specific ablation of a conditional IL-10 allele was induced by Cre recombinase knocked into the *Foxp3* gene locus (Rubtson et al., 2008). These mice were more prone to skin hypersensivity reaction induced by DNFB, thus formally demonstrating the implication of IL-10 in Treg mediated control of CHS.

Another potential mechanism through which Treg could inhibit effector migration to inflamed skin site, has been proposed by Ring and coworkers who found that Treg cell-derived adenosine plays a major role in preventing the elicitation of CHS reactions by blocking the interaction of effector T cells with the vascular endothelium (Ring et al., 2009).

Independently from the mechanism involved, CD4+CD25+Foxp3+ regulatory T cells require to be activated in order to develop their full suppressive capacity. Recently, studies from our and other groups better defined Treg activation in murine models of CHS. Analysing the expression kinetics of CD62L, CD69 and CD44 expression at Treg surface, Ring et al. showed that during the sensitization phase of CHS reactions, Treg get activated in the draining lymph nodes while Treg get activated in the blood during the elicitation phase. (Ring et aI., 2010). Employing the isolation protocol resumed in Fig. 4, we were able to extend the analysis of Treg activation to the skin tissue site in a model of primary allergic dermatitis (Simonetta et al., 2010). We confirmed that Treg were activated in lymph nodes after skin application of a strong hapten, as revealed by the surface upregulation of the activation molecules ICOS and CD103 (Fig. 5). Surprisingly when we extended the analysis to the skin tissue, we found high levels of ICOS and CD103 expression at surface of skin infiltrating Treg of both primed and non-primed animals (Fig. 5), indicating that skin Treg under normal physiological conditions are already in an activated state. A study performed by Vocanson and coworkers futher extended our results on ICOS expression on Treg revealing that these cells present superior suppressive activity and express IL-10, IL-17, and IFN-γ (Vocanson et al., 2010). More importantly for ACD comprehension, the authors showed that ICOS expressing Treg during ACD were hapten-specific, activated Treg cells proliferating in response to their cognate antigen in vivo.

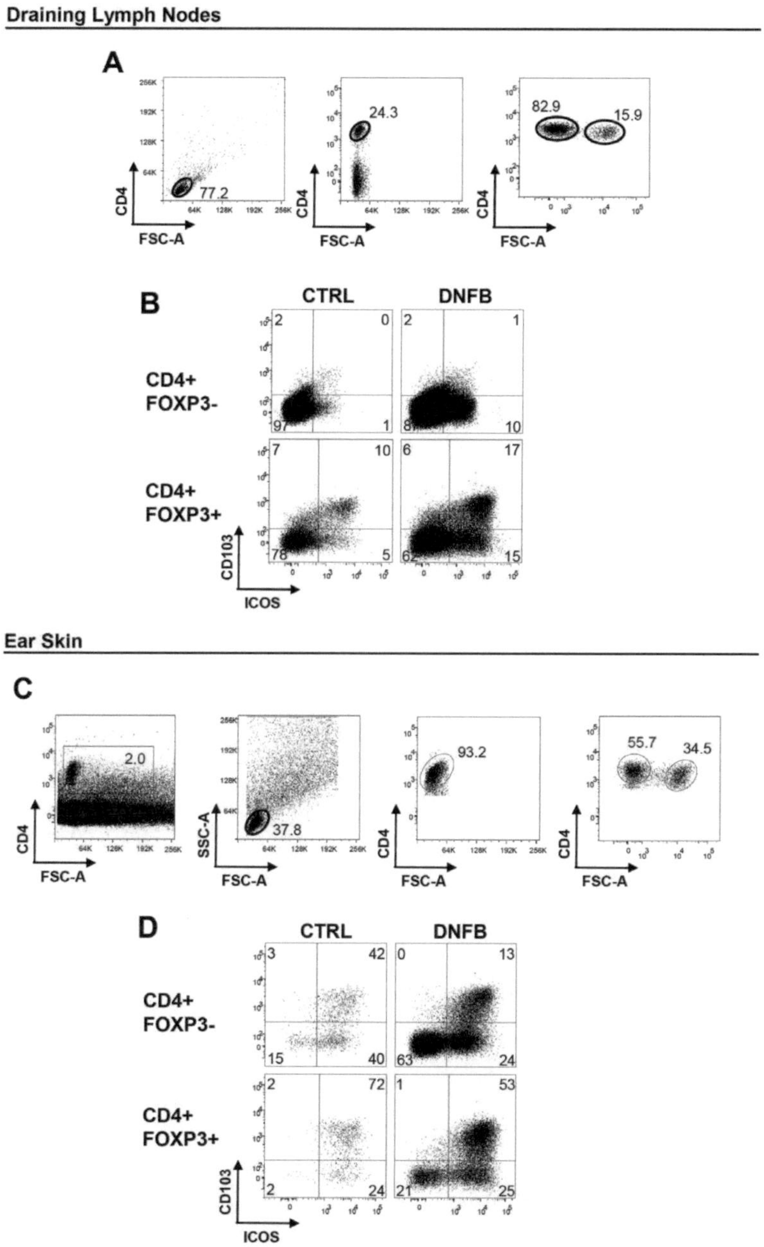

Fig. 5. FACS analysis of skin infiltrating CD4+ FOXP3+ Treg cells in a murine model of primary irritative contact dermatitis. (A, C) Gating strategy for Treg identification in draining lymph nodes (A) and ear skin (C). (B, D) ICOS and CD103 expression on CD4+FOXP3- conventional T cells and CD4+FOXP3+ Regulatory T cells from (B) draining lymph nodes and (D) ear skin. FSC-A, forward scatter; SSC-A, side scatter; CTRL, control.

6. Conclusions

Murine models of allergic and irritant skin inflammation have shed light into the pathogenesis of human contact dermatitis. They have highlighted the role of innate and adaptive immunity in allergic reactions to epicutaneously introduced allergens. More importantly, they allowed an in-depth dissection of cellular and molecular mechanisms involved in the development of the disease and will hopefully lead to new therapeutic interventions for this common dermatologic disorder.

7. Acknowledgements

This work was supported by the ANRS (Agence Nationale de la recherche contre le SIDA et les hepatites virales), Fondation Recherche Medicale (FRM) and Fondation de France.

8. References

Akiba H, Kehren J, Ducluzeau M-T, Krasteva M, Horand F, Kaiserlian D, Kaneko F & Nicolas J-F. (2002). Skin inflammation during contact hypersensitivity is mediated by early recruitment of CD8+ T cytotoxic 1 cells inducing keratinocyte apoptosis. *J. Immunol* Mar;168(6):3079-3087.

Antonopoulos C, Cumberbatch M, Dearman RJ, Daniel RJ, Kimber I & Groves RW. (2001). Functional caspase-1 is required for Langerhans cell migration and optimal contact sensitization in mice. *J. Immunol* Mar;166(6):3672-3677.

Antonopoulos C, Cumberbatch M, Mee JB, Dearman RJ, Wei X-Q, Liew FY, Kimber I, Groves RW. (2008). IL-18 is a key proximal mediator of contact hypersensitivity and allergen-induced Langerhans cell migration in murine epidermis. *J. Leukoc. Biol* Feb;83(2):361-367.

Bonneville M, Chavagnac C, Vocanson M, Rozieres A, Benetiere J, Pernet I, Denis A, Nicolas J-F, Hennino A. (2007). Skin contact irritation conditions the development and severity of allergic contact dermatitis. *J. Invest. Dermatol* Jun;127(6):1430-1435.

Bouloc A, Cavani A, Katz SI. (1998) Contact hypersensitivity in MHC class II-deficient mice depends on CD8 T lymphocytes primed by immunostimulating Langerhans cells. *J. Invest. Dermatol* Jul;111(1):44-49.

Bour H, Peyron E, Gaucherand M, Garrigue JL, Desvignes C, Kaiserlian D, Revillard JP, Nicolas JF. (1995). Major histocompatibility complex class I-restricted CD8+ T cells and class II-restricted CD4+ T cells, respectively, mediate and regulate contact sensitivity to dinitrofluorobenzene. *Eur. J. Immunol* Nov;25(11):3006-3010.

Cavani A, Nasorri F, Ottaviani C, Sebastiani S, De Pità O, Girolomoni G. (2003). Human CD25+ regulatory T cells maintain immune tolerance to nickel in healthy, nonallergic individuals. *J. Immunol* Dec;171(11):5760-5768.

Cumberbatch M, Dearman RJ, Groves RW, Antonopoulos C, Kimber I. (2002). Differential regulation of epidermal langerhans cell migration by interleukins (IL)-1alpha and IL-1beta during irritant- and allergen-induced cutaneous immune responses. *Toxicol. Appl. Pharmacol* Jul;182(2):126-135.

Desvignes C, Bour H, Nicolas JF, Kaiserlian D. (1996) Lack of oral tolerance but oral priming for contact sensitivity to dinitrofluorobenzene in major histocompatibility complex class II-deficient mice and in CD4+ T cell-depleted mice. *Eur. J. Immunol* Aug;26(8):1756-1761.

Desvignes C, Etchart N, Kehren J, Akiba I, Nicolas JF, Kaiserlian D. (2000) Oral administration of hapten inhibits in vivo induction of specific cytotoxic CD8+ T cells mediating tissue inflammation: a role for regulatory CD4+ T cells. *J. Immunol* Mar;164(5):2515-2522.

Dubois B, Chapat L, Goubier A, Papiernik M, Nicolas J-F, Kaiserlian D. (2003). Innate CD4+CD25+ regulatory T cells are required for oral tolerance and inhibition of CD8+ T cells mediating skin inflammation. *Blood* Nov;102(9):3295-3301.

Eisen HN, Orris L, Belman S. (1952). Elicitation of delayed allergic skin reactions with haptens; the dependence of elicitation on hapten combination with protein. *J. Exp. Med* May;95(5):473-487.

Enk AH, Angeloni VL, Udey MC, Katz SI. (1993). An essential role for Langerhans cell-derived IL-1 beta in the initiation of primary immune responses in skin. *J. Immunol* May;150(9):3698-3704.

Fontenot JD, Gavin MA, Rudensky AY. (2003). Foxp3 programs the development and function of CD4+CD25+ regulatory T cells. *Nat. Immunol* Apr;4(4):330-336.

Gocinski BL, Tigelaar RE. (1990). Roles of CD4+ and CD8+ T cells in murine contact sensitivity revealed by in vivo monoclonal antibody depletion. *J. Immunol* Jun;144(11):4121-4128.[cited 2011 Jul 7]

He D, Wu L, Kim HK, Li H, Elmets CA, Xu H. *(2006)* CD8+ IL-17-producing T cells are important in effector functions for the elicitation of contact hypersensitivity responses. *J. Immunol* Nov;177(10):6852-6858.

Kanerva L, Tarvainen K, Pinola A, Leino T, Granlund H, Estlander T, Jolanki R, Förström L. (1994). A single accidental exposure may result in a chemical burn, primary sensitization and allergic contact dermatitis. *Contact Derm* Oct;31(4):229-235.

Kehren J, Desvignes C, Krasteva M, Ducluzeau MT, Assossou O, Horand F, Hahne M, Kägi D, Kaiserlian D, Nicolas JF. (1999) Cytotoxicity is mandatory for CD8(+) T cell-mediated contact hypersensitivity. *J. Exp. Med* Mar;189(5):779-786.

Kish DD, Gorbachev AV, Fairchild RL. (2005). CD8+ T cells produce IL-2, which is required for CD(4+)CD25+ T cell regulation of effector CD8+ T cell development for contact hypersensitivity responses. *J. Leukoc. Biol* Sep;78(3):725-735.

Klekotka PA, Yang L, Yokoyama WM. (2010). Contrasting roles of the IL-1 and IL-18 receptors in MyD88-dependent contact hypersensitivity. *J. Invest. Dermatol* Jan;130(1):184-191.

Kohler J, Martin S, Pflugfelder U, Ruh H, Vollmer J, Weltzien HU. (1995) Cross-reactive trinitrophenylated peptides as antigens for class II major histocompatibility complex-restricted T cells and inducers of contact sensitivity in mice. Limited T cell receptor repertoire. *Eur. J. Immunol* Jan;25(1):92-101.

Kondo S, Pastore S, Fujisawa H, Shivji GM, McKenzie RC, Dinarello CA, Sauder DN. (1995). Interleukin-1 receptor antagonist suppresses contact hypersensitivity. *J. Invest. Dermatol* Sep;105(3):334-338.

Krasteva M, Kehren J, Horand F, Akiba H, Choquet G, Ducluzeau MT, Tédone R, Garrigue JL, Kaiserlian D, Nicolas JF. (1998). Dual role of dendritic cells in the induction and down-regulation of antigen-specific cutaneous inflammation. *J. Immunol* Feb;160(3):1181-1190.

Kripke ML, Munn CG, Jeevan A, Tang JM, Bucana C. (1990). Evidence that cutaneous antigen-presenting cells migrate to regional lymph nodes during contact sensitization. *J. Immunol* Nov;145(9):2833-2838.

Lu B, Ebensperger C, Dembic Z, Wang Y, Kvatyuk M, Lu T, Coffman RL, Pestka S, Rothman PB. (1998). Targeted disruption of the interferon-gamma receptor 2 gene results in severe immune defects in mice. *Proc. Natl. Acad. Sci. U.S.A* Jul;95(14):8233-8238.

Martin S, Lappin MB, Kohler J, Delattre V, Leicht C, Preckel T, Simon JC, Weltzien HU. (2000). Peptide immunization indicates that CD8+ T cells are the dominant effector cells in trinitrophenyl-specific contact hypersensitivity. *J. Invest. Dermatol* Aug;115(2):260-266.

Martin SF, Dudda JC, Bachtanian E, Lembo A, Liller S, Dürr C, Heimesaat MM, Bereswill S, Fejer G, Vassileva R, Jakob T, Freudenberg N, Termeer CC, Johner C, Galanos C, Freudenberg MA. Toll-like receptor and IL-12 signaling control susceptibility to contact hypersensitivity. J. Exp. Med 2008 Sep;205(9):2151-2162.

Miller SD, Jenkins MK. In vivo effects of GK1.5 (anti-L3T4a) monoclonal antibody on induction and expression of delayed-type hypersensitivity. Cell. Immunol 1985 May;92(2):414-426.

Moorhead JW. Tolerance and contact sensitivity to DNFA in mice. VIII. Identification of distinct T cell subpopulations that mediate in vivo and in vitro manifestations of delayed hypersensitivity. J. Immunol 1978 Jan;120(1):137-144.

Naik SM, Cannon G, Burbach GJ, Singh SR, Swerlick RA, Wilcox JN, Ansel JC, Caughman SW. Human keratinocytes constitutively express interleukin-18 and secrete biologically active interleukin-18 after treatment with pro-inflammatory mediators and dinitrochlorobenzene. J. Invest. Dermatol 1999 Nov;113(5):766-772.

Nakae S, Komiyama Y, Nambu A, Sudo K, Iwase M, Homma I, Sekikawa K, Asano M, Iwakura Y. (2002). Antigen-specific T cell sensitization is impaired in IL-17-deficient mice, causing suppression of allergic cellular and humoral responses. *Immunity* Sep;17(3):375-387.

Reeve VE, Bosnic M, Nishimura N. (1999). Interferon-gamma is involved in photoimmunoprotection by UVA (320-400 nm) radiation in mice. *J. Invest. Dermatol* Jun;112(6):945-950.

Ring S, Enk AH, Mahnke K. (2010) ATP activates regulatory T Cells in vivo during contact hypersensitivity reactions. *J. Immunol* Apr;184(7):3408-3416.

Ring S, Karakhanova S, Johnson T, Enk AH, Mahnke K. (2010). Gap junctions between regulatory T cells and dendritic cells prevent sensitization of CD8(+) T cells. *J. Allergy Clin. Immunol* Jan;125(1):237-246.e1-7.

Ring S, Oliver SJ, Cronstein BN, Enk AH, Mahnke K. (2009). CD4+CD25+ regulatory T cells suppress contact hypersensitivity reactions through a CD39, adenosine-dependent mechanism. *J. Allergy Clin. Immunol* Jun;123(6):1287-1296.e2.

Ring S, Schäfer SC, Mahnke K, Lehr H-A, Enk AH. (2006). CD4+ CD25+ regulatory T cells suppress contact hypersensitivity reactions by blocking influx of effector T cells into inflamed tissue. *Eur. J. Immunol* Nov;36(11):2981-2992.

Rückert R, Brandt K, Hofmann U, Bulfone-Paus S, Paus R. (2002). IL-2-IgG2b fusion protein suppresses murine contact hypersensitivity in vivo. *J. Invest. Dermatol* Aug;119(2):370-376.[cited 2011 Jul 7]

Saint-Mezard P, Krasteva M, Chavagnac C, Bosset S, Akiba H, Kehren J, Kanitakis J, Kaiserlian D, Nicolas JF, Berard F. (2003). Afferent and efferent phases of allergic contact dermatitis (ACD) can be induced after a single skin contact with haptens: evidence using a mouse model of primary ACD. *J. Invest. Dermatol* Apr;120(4):641-647.

Saint-Mezard P, Berard F, Dubois B, Kaiserlian D, Nicolas J-F. (2004) The role of CD4+ and CD8+ T cells in contact hypersensitivity and allergic contact dermatitis. *Eur J Dermatol* Jun;14(3):131-138.

Saint-Mezard P, Chavagnac C, Vocanson M, Kehren J, Rozières A, Bosset S, Ionescu M, Dubois B, Kaiserlian D, Nicolas J-F, Bérard F. (2005). Deficient contact hypersensitivity reaction in CD4-/- mice is because of impaired hapten-specific CD8+ T cell functions. *J. Invest. Dermatol* Mar;124(3):562-569.

Sakaguchi S, Sakaguchi N, Asano M, Itoh M, Toda M. (1995) Immunologic self-tolerance maintained by activated T cells expressing IL-2 receptor alpha-chains (CD25). Breakdown of a single mechanism of self-tolerance causes various autoimmune diseases. *J. Immunol* Aug;155(3):1151-1164.

Sakaguchi S, Yamaguchi T, Nomura T, Ono M. (2008). Regulatory T cells and immune tolerance. *Cell* May;133(5):775-787.

Sauder DN, Dinarello CA, Morhenn VB. (1984). Langerhans cell production of interleukin-1. *J. Invest. Dermatol* 1984 Jun;82(6):605-607.

Saulnier M, Huang S, Aguet M, Ryffel B. (1995). Role of interferon-gamma in contact hypersensitivity assessed in interferon-gamma receptor-deficient mice. *Toxicology* Sep;102(3):301-312.

Shornick LP, De Togni P, Mariathasan S, Goellner J, Strauss-Schoenberger J, Karr RW, Ferguson TA, Chaplin DD. (1996). Mice deficient in IL-1beta manifest impaired contact hypersensitivity to trinitrochlorobenzone. *J. Exp. Med* Apr;183(4):1427-1436.

Simonetta F, Chiali A, Cordier C, Urrutia A, Girault I, Bloquet S, Tanchot C, Bourgeois C. (2010) Increased CD127 expression on activated FOXP3+CD4+ regulatory T cells. *Eur. J. Immunol* Sep;40(9):2528-2538.

Sutterwala FS, Ogura Y, Szczepanik M, Lara-Tejero M, Lichtenberger GS, Grant EP, Bertin J, Coyle AJ, Galán JE, Askenase PW, Flavell RA. (2006). Critical role for NALP3/CIAS1/Cryopyrin in innate and adaptive immunity through its regulation of caspase-1. *Immunity* Mar;24(3):317-327.

van Loveren H, Meade R, Askenase PW. (1983). An early component of delayed-type hypersensitivity mediated by T cells and mast cells. *J. Exp. Med* May;157(5):1604-1617.

Vocanson M, Hennino A, Cluzel-Tailhardat M, Saint-Mezard P, Benetiere J, Chavagnac C, Berard F, Kaiserlian D, Nicolas J-F. (2006). CD8+ T cells are effector cells of contact dermatitis to common skin allergens in mice. *J. Invest. Dermatol* Apr;126(4):815-820.

Vocanson M, Hennino A, Rozières A, Cluzel-Tailhardat M, Poyet G, Valeyrie M, Bénetière J, Tédone R, Kaiserlian D, Nicolas J-F. (2009). Skin exposure to weak and moderate contact allergens induces IFNgamma production by lymph node cells of CD4+ T-cell-depleted mice. *J. Invest. Dermatol* May;129(5):1185-1191.

Vocanson M, Rozieres A, Hennino A, Poyet G, Gaillard V, Renaudineau S, Achachi A, Benetiere J, Kaiserlian D, Dubois B, Nicolas J-F. (2010). Inducible costimulator (ICOS) is a marker for highly suppressive antigen-specific T cells sharing features of TH17/TH1 and regulatory T cells. *J. Allergy Clin. Immunol* Aug;126(2):280-289, 289.e1-7.

Wang B, Fujisawa H, Zhuang L, Freed I, Howell BG, Shahid S, Shivji GM, Mak TW, Sauder DN. (2000) CD4+ Th1 and CD8+ type 1 cytotoxic T cells both play a crucial role in the full development of contact hypersensitivity. *J. Immunol* Dec;165(12):6783-6790.

Wang B, Feliciani C, Howell BG, Freed I, Cai Q, Watanabe H, Sauder DN. (2002). Contribution of Langerhans cell-derived IL-18 to contact hypersensitivity. *J. Immunol* Apr;168(7):3303-3308.

Watanabe H, Gaide O, Pétrilli V, Martinon F, Contassot E, Roques S, Kummer JA, Tschopp J, French LE. (2007). Activation of the IL-1beta-processing inflammasome is involved in contact hypersensitivity. *J. Invest. Dermatol* Aug;127(8):1956-1963.

Weltzien HU, Moulon C, Martin S, Padovan E, Hartmann U, Kohler J. (1996). T cell immune responses to haptens. Structural models for allergic and autoimmune reactions. *Toxicology* Feb;107(2):141-151.

Xu H, DiIulio NA, Fairchild RL. (1996) T cell populations primed by hapten sensitization in contact sensitivity are distinguished by polarized patterns of cytokine production: interferon gamma-producing (Tc1) effector CD8+ T cells and interleukin (Il) 4/Il-10-producing (Th2) negative regulatory CD4+ T cells. *J. Exp. Med* Mar;183(3):1001-1012.

3

Keratinocytes, Innate Immunity and Allergic Contact Dermatitis - Opportunities for the Development of *In Vitro* Assays to Predict the Sensitizing Potential of Chemicals

Jochem W. van der Veen[1,2], Rob J. Vandebriel[2],
Henk van Loveren[1,2] and Janine Ezendam[2]
[1]*Maastricht University, Department of Toxicogenomics, The Netherlands*
[2]*National Institute for Public Health and the Environment, The Netherlands*

1. Introduction

Allergic contact dermatitis (ACD) is the most prevalent form of immunotoxicity in humans characterized by clinical manifestations such as red rashes, itchy skin and blisters. The disease is caused by skin sensitizers which are allergenic low-molecular weight chemicals. ACD is an important occupational disease that gives problems at different workplaces, including hair dressers, metal workers, construction workers, and cleaners. In addition, ACD can develop in the general population as well, since several consumer products contain skin sensitizers. Important skin sensitizers are metals (nickel, chromium), fragrances, hair dye ingredients and preservatives (Kimber et al., 2002a; Vandebriel & van Loveren, 2010).

ACD is a typical type IV (delayed-type) hypersensitivity response that develops in two phases, the initiation phase in which the immune system is sensitized and the elicitation phase in which the clinical symptoms develop. At initiation, the low-molecular weight and polarity of skin sensitizers allow for penetration of the stratum corneum of the skin. In addition, protein reactivity is a hallmark of skin sensitizers. After binding to proteins in the skin, hapten-carrier complexes are formed (Kimber et al., 2002a; Berard et al., 2003; Vandebriel & van Loveren, 2010). The formation of these hapten-protein complexes is crucial, since the chemicals themselves are not immunogenic and priming of T cells can only occur after formation of these complexes. After taking up these hapten-carrier complexes, immature Langerhans cells and dendritic cells start to migrate to the draining lymph node and become potent T cell activators through the upregulation of costimulatory molecules (Gaspari, 1997; Kimber et al., 2002a; Berard et al., 2003; Vocanson et al., 2009; Vandebriel & van Loveren, 2010). Hapten specific T cells are activated through a combination of haptenized peptide presentation on major histocompatibility complex (MHC) molecules and costimulatory molecules, such as CD54, CD80 and CD86. Activated T cells undergo clonal expansion, thereby generating skin homing CD8+ Tc1/Tc17 and CD4+ Th1/Th17 effector T cells that enter the blood circulation (Kimber et al., 2002a; Freudenberg et al., 2009 ; Vocanson et al., 2009; Vandebriel & van Loveren, 2010). After being sensitized, subsequent skin contact with the hapten will elicit skin symptoms within 48 hours caused by the hapten specific T cells that migrate into the skin. Here they recognize the protein/hapten complex presented by either dendritic cells or keratinocytes. Upon recognition, the T cells become activated and start to produce typical Th1 and Th17 response cytokines, such as IFN-γ, IL-12, IL-17, and IL-23 (Kimber & Dearman, 2002; Zhao et al., 2009).

The identification of chemicals with skin sensitizing capacity is of great importance to ensure the safety of industrial chemicals and cosmetic ingredients. The current testing methods for skin sensitization are animal tests, either using guinea pigs (Guinea Pig Maximization Test or the Buehler Test) or mice (the murine Local Lymph Node Assay) (Kimber et al., 1994; Gerberick et al., 2007a). Recently, the pressure to develop non-animal testing strategies has increased due to public and political influence. The 7th amendment to the European Union (EU) Cosmetics Directive forbids the use of animal tests and the sensitizing potential of a great number of chemicals will have to be evaluated within the framework of Registration, Evaluation, Authorization and Restriction of Chemical substances (REACH). Therefore, there is a great demand for in vitro alternative test methods that can replace the currently used animal assays. Knowledge on physical-chemical properties of haptens together with insight in the immunological mechanisms that lead to sensitization need to be applied in the alternative methods that are currently being developed or validated. The elucidation of pathways that play a role in the initiation phase of skin sensitization have long been subject of investigations. Several *in vitro* and *in vivo* studies have shown that pathways linked to innate immunity and oxidative stress are important in the first phase of skin sensitization (Natsch, 2009; Vandebriel et al., 2010; Martin et al., 2011). Activation of these pathways induces cell stress and damage, and production of pro-inflammatory cytokines and chemokines. In this way, 'danger' signals are produced in the skin, which are considered to be required for further development of an adaptive immune response (Kimber et al., 2002b; Martin et al., 2011).

In the skin, keratinocytes are abundantly present and these cells are the first to encounter haptens that penetrate through the skin. Keratinocytes are considered to be key players in the initiation phase of skin sensitization for several reasons (Figure 1). Keratinocytes contain enzymes with metabolic activity required for the conversion of prohaptens into biologically active haptens, thereby facilitating binding to proteins (Van Pelt et al., 1990; Gelardi et al., 2001). In addition, keratinocytes have been shown to express chemotactic factors upon exposure to sensitizers, including chemokines (CXCL8, CXCL9, CXCL10, CXCL11) and adhesion molecules (ICAM-1). These attract more immune cells to the exposed skin area, thereby strengthening the immune response (Gaspari, 1997; Albanesi, 2010). Keratinocytes are important in the elicitation phase of ACD as well, since they are able to present antigen to the surroundings through both MHC class I and MHC class II molecules (Albanesi et al., 2005; Nestle et al., 2009). In addition, after being targeted by IFN-γ, keratinocytes upregulate costimulatory molecules such as CD80 and are able to function as antigen presenting cells and facilitating activation of hapten specific T cells (Gaspari, 1997; Albanesi, 2010). Hence, keratinocytes are important in the sensitization and elicitation phase of ACD and for that reason these cells are often used for the development of *in vitro* assays for skin sensitization testing (Van Och et al., 2005; Corsini et al., 2009; Vandebriel et al., 2010; Galbiati et al., 2011).

In the development of *in vitro* assays, human keratinocyte cell lines, primary keratinocytes, and 3D skin models are used. In order to base read-outs of these assays on toxicological relevant pathways it is important to understand the underlying mechanisms of skin sensitization. In this chapter, an overview of current knowledge on the role of innate immune and oxidative stress pathways in skin sensitization will be provided together with the relevance of these pathways for the development of *in vitro* assays using keratinocytes.

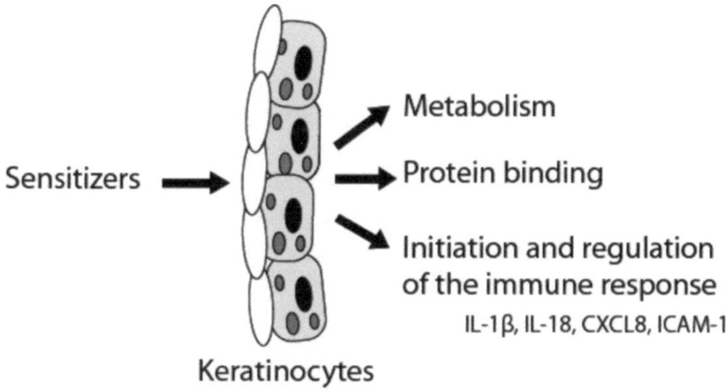

Fig. 1. Keratinocyte responses to sensitizers

2. Innate immune responses: Toll-like receptors and other pattern recognition receptors

The induction of innate signaling pathways by skin sensitizers in keratinocytes is believed to be a crucial factor in skin sensitization and a requirement for activation of Langerhans cells and dendritic cells and subsequent T cell priming (Martin et al., 2011). Studies have demonstrated that human primary keratinocytes express mRNA for Toll-like receptors (TLRs), such as TLR 1, 2, 3, 4, 5 and 9 (Kollisch et al., 2005; Son et al., 2006), which are important receptors of the innate immune system. Upon TLR activation, keratinocytes are able to produce a range of cytokines and chemokines, which allows for attraction of other immune cells, such as dendritic cells (Lebre et al., 2007).

TLRs are the first family to be identified of the germ-line encoded pattern recognition receptors (PRR). These receptors are involved in the first line of defense against pathogens. To date, 10 different TLRs have been identified in humans (Boehme & Compton, 2004). The TLRs are known to recognize various pathogen associated molecular patterns (PAMPs), which are conserved and essential molecules of pathogens. Some well-known examples are lipopolysaccharide (LPS) that is recognized by TLR4, double-stranded RNA recognized by TLR3 and lipopeptides recognized by TLR2 (Hosogi et al., 2004; Lebre et al., 2007; Kumar et al., 2009). The primary function of TLRs is the initial recognition of pathogenic microorganisms and subsequent activation of the innate immune response. Most pathogens express multiple PAMPs and are thus recognized by multiple TLRs. Activated TLRs will promote the phagocytosis of pathogens in innate immune cells such as macrophages and induce a respiratory burst, production of ROS and RNS, to neutralize pathogens. Combined, this promotes the presentation of pathogen specific peptides to cells of the adaptive immune system. Furthermore, the secreted reactive oxygen species can act as signaling molecules and have been identified to be important pro-inflammatory mediators. Upon TLR activation, cells start to produce pro-inflammatory cytokines, attracting more immune cells to the site of infection (Kawai & Akira, 2009). In addition, TLRs are able to recognize endogenous danger signals, known as danger-associated molecular patterns (DAMPs). These molecules are released under cellular stress and include components of the extracellular matrix, such as hyaluronic acid and biglycan, heat shock proteins and uric acid crystals (Seong & Matzinger, 2004; Wheeler et al., 2009; Kawai & Akira, 2010; Martin et al., 2011).

Another important family of pattern recognition receptors are the nucleotide-binding oligomerization domain (NOD)-like receptors (NLRs). These intracellular receptors recognize PAMPs with the same leucine-rich repeat domains that can be found in TLRs. NLRs are activated by PAMPs such as bacterial RNA, flagellin and breakdown products of peptidoglycan (Feldmeyer et al., 2010). In addition, the NLRs are able to recognize DAMPs such as ATP and uric acid (Kawai & Akira, 2009). Upon activation, NOD receptors can activate NF-κB and large protein complexes called inflammasomes (Stutz et al., 2009; Feldmeyer et al., 2010; Latz, 2010). The inflammasomes are required to activate and secrete several cytokines that are expressed as nonfunctional proteins after NF-κB activation. The most important of these are IL-1β and IL-18, which are expressed as pro-IL-1β and pro-IL-18, respectively (Nestle et al., 2009).

2.1 Mechanisms of TLR activation

Several TLRs are located at the cell membrane, while others are in endosomal membranes (Figure 2). All TLRs consist of three domains: a leucine rich repeat domain that recognizes PAMPs, an anchoring transmembrane domain and a cytoplasmatic Toll/interleukin-1 receptor (TIR) domain involved in signal transduction (Kumar et al., 2009; Olaru & Jensen, 2010). Adaptor proteins need to bind to the TIR domain to ensure continuation and amplification of the signal transduction. The majority of TLRs use the myeloid differentiation primary-response gene 88 (MyD88) as adaptor, except TLR3 which uses the TIR-domain containing adaptor protein inducing IFN-β (TRIF). TLR4 can use both MyD88 and TRIF for signal transduction, with MyD88 being involved in the majority of TLR4 mediated processes (Hosogi et al., 2004; Lebre et al., 2007; Trinchieri & Sher, 2007; Kumar et al., 2009).

Through PAMP recognition, the TLRs homodimerize and enable the binding of the adaptor protein. An exception is the TLR2 molecule which forms heterodimers with either TLR1 or TLR6. Following activation of the MyD88 adaptor protein, a signaling cascade involving mitogen-activated protein kinases (MAPK) and ending with the ubiquitination of IκB occurs. This induces the release of NF-κB, resulting in the transcription of pro-inflammatory cytokines such as IFN-α, IL1-β and CXCL8. After activation of TRIF the resulting signaling cascade ends with the activation of IFN regulatory factors (IRFs) and the induction of type I IFNs. The expression pattern differs for each TLR. The activation of TLR3 by poly I:C generally leads to the production of the largest panel of cytokines and chemokines, including CCL2, CCL20, CCL27, CXCL8, CXCL9, CXCL10, and TNF-α. In comparison, activation of TLR4 using LPS leads to the production of CCL2, CCL20, CXCL8, and TNF-α (Lebre et al., 2007; Olaru & Jensen, 2010).

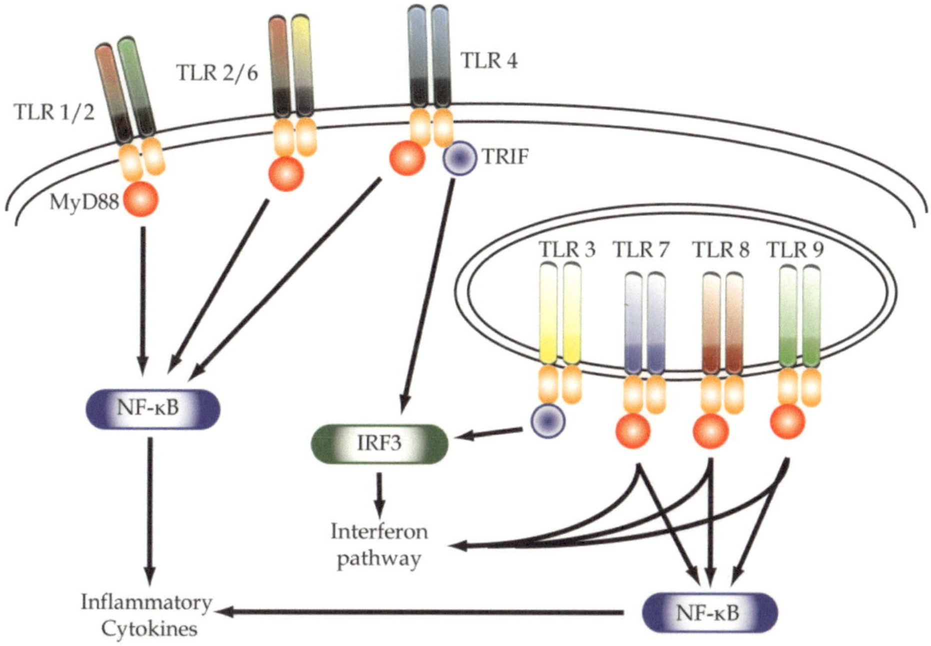

Fig. 2. Schematic presentation of TLR localization and signaling pathways (Boehme & Compton, 2004). TLR2 in combination with either TLR1 or TLR6, as well as TLR4, are expressed on the cell surface and use MyD88 as adaptor for cell signaling. This leads to NF-κB activation and inflammatory cytokine secretion. In addition to MyD88, TLR4 uses TRIF to activate IRF3 and the IFN pathway. TLRs 3, 7, 8, and 9 typically localize to endosomal membranes, where they detect a variety of nucleic acids. TLR3 utilizes TRIF to activate IRF3. TLRs 7, 8, and 9 trigger inflammatory cytokine secretion and the IFN pathway through MyD88.

3. The role of TLRs in skin sensitization

The importance of TLRs in skin sensitization has been shown *in vivo* by using different types of TLR knockout mice. In the majority of these experiments, the ear swelling response was measured as a read-out for contact hypersensitivity responses. Mice deficient of TLR2 had reduced ear swelling after challenge with the skin sensitizer oxazolone and these mice were unable to launch an effector Th1 response (Jin et al., 2009). The importance of TLR2 in skin sensitization was confirmed by Martin et al (2008), showing a reduced ear swelling in response to the skin sensitizers trinitrochlorobenzene (TNCB), oxazolone and fluorescein isothiocyanate (FITC). Skin sensitization to these compounds was completely prevented in the combined absence of TLR2 and TLR4, indicating that for full induction of sensitization both TLRs are required (Martin et al., 2008). More evidence for the importance of TLRs in skin sensitization was found in experiments in mice deficient for the TLR adaptor molecule MyD88. These mice were unable to mount an ear swelling response to dinitrofluorobenzene (DNFB), which was explained by an impaired upregulation of CD86 on dendritic cells, leading to a reduced activation of hapten specific T cells. In contrast, mice lacking TLR2, TLR4, TLR6 or TLR9 had no impaired ear swelling in response to DNFB. Mice deficient of the adaptor molecule TRIF could be sensitized to DNFB, indicating that TLR3, using only TRIF for signal transduction, is not involved in skin sensitization (Klekotka et al., 2010).

More evidence for the importance of TLR in skin sensitization has recently been found for nickel, one of the most prevalent human sensitizers. Remarkably, nickel is a false-negative in the mouse LLNA. This paradox was recently explained by the discovery that nickel interacts directly with non-conserved histidine residues in human but not mouse TLR4, thereby activating the innate immune system and driving the development of ACD (Schmidt et al., 2010). Taken together, these data show that especially TLR 2 and 4 play an important role in mounting a full immune response to skin sensitizers.

Evidence for an involvement of the signaling pathway p38 MAPK in skin sensitization further underpin the relevance for TLR. p38 MAPK are enzymes that play an important role in the signal transduction of TLR (Mehrotra et al., 2007). In mice treated with the specific p38 MAPK inhibitor SB202190 the ear swelling in response to DNFB was impaired (Takanami-Ohnishi et al., 2002). Further evidence for the importance of p38 MAPK was found in *in vitro* studies. In dendritic cells exposed to DNFB, DNCB or nickel, the signaling pathways p38 MAPK and extracellular signal-regulated kinase (ERK) were activated (Matos et al., 2005; Miyazawa et al., 2008). In the keratinocyte cell line NCTC2544 IL-18 production induced by skin sensitizers was greatly decreased after addition of a specific p38 MAPK inhibitor, SB203580 (Galbiati et al., 2011). Similar results were obtained in an experiment using the monocytic THP-1 cell line (Mitjans et al., 2010). These signaling pathways are essential for the further maturation of dendritic cells and the activation of hapten-specific T cells, since they trigger the production of cytokines such as TNF-α, IL-6, IL-12 and IL-18 in keratinocytes or dendritic cells and are essential in the upregulation of costimulatory molecules on the surface of the dendritic cells (Antonios et al., 2009; Antonios et al., 2010).

It is not clear which ligands trigger TLR activation after exposure to skin sensitizers. It has been shown that ACD can develop in germ-free mice; hence danger signals from pathogenic microbes are not required for sensitization. This indicates that the presence of haptens is sufficient for TLR activation and presumably endogenous TLR ligands are involved (Martin et al., 2008). Several endogenous danger signals can be formed by the breakdown of extracellular matrix under influence of oxidative stress induced by sensitizers. These fragments can be recognized by TLR and initiate the innate immune response. In addition, NF-κB regulates hyaluronidases that degrade hyaluronic acid. Transcription of these enzymes can therefore be a result of earlier TLR activation, eventually strengthening the TLR activation in the skin (Martin et al., 2011). Another possible endogenous danger signal is uric acid, which can be released due to damage to the skin. Mice that were exposed to a combination of TNCB, uric acid crystals and an uricase inhibitor have increased sensitization. Uric acid has been shown to activate the NLRP3 inflammasome, thereby facilitating cytokine production (Liu et al., 2007). Other endogenous danger signals that have been linked to skin sensitization include the heat-shock proteins 27 and 70, which are also recognized by TLR4. Neutralizing antibodies for these heat shock proteins resulted in an impaired ear swelling in response to DNFB. In addition, the cytokine profile shifted from a Th1 to a Th2 repertoire (Yusuf et al., 2009).

3.1 The role of Nod-like receptors and the inflammasome in skin sensitization

TLRs are not the only PRR family members that play a role in the development of ACD, NOD-Like receptors (NLR) have also been implicated, especially their ability to form or activate inflammasomes containing caspase-1 is important. Ear swelling responses to DNFB or oxazolone were decreased significantly in caspase-1 knock out mice when compared to wild type mice (Antonopoulos et al., 2001). In addition, migration of Langerhans cells was evaluated in wildtype and caspase-1 deficient mice. It was shown that in the absence of caspase-1 the migration of Langerhans cells was impaired, but the maturation of Langerhans cells was not affected. In these mice, Langerhans cells migration could be restored when IL1-β, but not TNF-α were intradermally injected, indicating that these mice were unable to produce IL1-β, which is dependent on caspase-1 (Antonopoulos et al., 2001; Cumberbatch et al., 2001). IL1-α has been shown to have a marked effect on skin sensitization as well, since ear swelling in response to TNBS was impaired in IL1-α deficient mice and not in IL1-β deficient mice (Nakae et al., 2001). Whereas IL1-β is mainly produced by Langerhans cells, keratinocytes are the main source of IL1-α. These studies show that IL1-α is required in the induction of skin sensitization, whereas IL1-β plays an important role in Langerhans migration.

The NLRP3 inflammasome can be assembled due to the activation of the $P2X_7$ receptor. This receptor on the cell membrane recognizes extracellular ATP, which is a damage-associated molecular pattern. Mice deficient of $P2X_7$ had impaired ear swelling responses after exposure to TNCB and oxazolone. The ear swelling response was restored when a potent $P2X_7$-independent NLRP3 activator was applied. To determine whether the triggering of NLRP3 via $P2X_7$ is specific to sensitizers remains to be determined (Weber et al., 2010).

Importantly, the activation of inflammasomes seems to be an effect that is not specific to sensitizers. Other chemicals, such as irritants can also induce cellular stress and activate the inflammasome. The same stress that causes activation of inflammasomes could also lead to the degradation of hyaluronic acid and thus activation of TLR. Hence, this illustrates that NLRP3 inflammasome activation is not limited to skin sensitization and that this pathway cannot be used for the identification of skin sensitizing properties.

3.2 Effects of co-exposure to PAMPs on skin sensitization

In the initiation of skin sensitization, innate immune responses play an important role and it has been shown that skin sensitizers are able to trigger this pathway via PRR members. In reality it is possible that humans with an existing skin inflammation are exposed to haptens. This inflammation leads to microbial danger signals in the skin which could possibly aggravate the immune response induced by skin sensitizers. Evidence for this was found in *in vivo* studies in which the effects of PAMPs on ACD development were studied in mice using TLR4, 7 and 9 ligands.

In C57BL6 and C3H/HeN mice that were prior to sensitization exposed to the TLR4 ligand LPS by intradermal ear injection the ear swelling response to DNFB was increased. In the TLR4 deficient C3H/HeJ strain, co-exposure with LPS did not enhance the ear swelling response, providing evidence for a crucial role of TLR4 activation (Yokoi et al., 2009). The dose required for sensitization to DNFB was reduced a 100-fold when mice were pretreated with R-848, a TLR7 ligand (Gunzer et al., 2005). Pretreatment with the TLR9 ligand CpG ODN enhanced ear swelling in response to DNFB, but it was shown that the site of exposure to CpG ODN is important. When the site of hapten exposure was not the same as the CpG administration site, no effect on skin sensitization was observed, illustrating that co-existing inflammatory signaling in the same skin area is needed to enhance the response (Akiba et al., 2004). There is evidence that a reduced skin barrier function, caused by mutations in the filaggrin gene, increases the sensitization rates to nickel (Novak et al., 2008; Metz & Maurer, 2009). Possibly, the impaired barrier function leads to more pathogen exposure and increased TLR activation. On the other hand, this mutation might also lead to increased skin penetration of the haptens thereby increasing the bioavailability in the skin.

In general, when mice are exposed to a hapten together with PAMPs, the ACD response is enhanced, which is most likely due to the increased activation of the innate immune system. In the skin, multiple danger signals are produced in response to the PAMPs thereby facilitating the innate immune response and subsequent adaptive immune response. Therefore, it is possible that concurrent hapten and pathogen exposure leads to increased risk of sensitization.

4. The role of the Nrf2-KEAP1 pathway in skin sensitization

Besides triggering the innate immune response, *in vitro* studies have shown that exposure to skin sensitizers induced oxidative stress in keratinocytes and dendritic cells (Matsue et al., 2003; Mehrotra et al., 2005). Particularly the antioxidant response Nuclear factor (erythroid-derived 2)-like 2 (Nrf2)-Keap1 pathway has been identified to play an important role in sensitization. The importance of this pathway has been shown in several microarray studies, in which gene expression analysis revealed that genes downstream of Nrf2 were highly upregulated in sensitizer exposed keratinocytes and dendritic cells (Ade et al., 2009; Python et al., 2009; Vandebriel et al., 2010). The relevance of Nrf2 for skin sensitization has been shown in Nrf2 deficient mice. The ear swelling in response to DNFB and oxazolone was reduced but not completely prevented in old (but not young) Nrf2 deficient mice. Furthermore, in these old mice it was shown that IFN-γ but not IL-4 production was absent, indicating that Nrf2 plays a role in the type 1 T cell response (Kim et al., 2008).

Under physiological conditions, the transcription factor (Nrf2) is bound to the sensory protein Keap1 (Figure 3). This complex promotes Cul-3 mediated ubiquitination and subsequent degradation of Nrf2. In response to oxidative stress, the highly reactive Cys residues of Keap1 are activated and Nrf2 is released (Niture et al., 2009). The free Nrf2 translocates into the nucleus and forms a complex with small MAF (F, G and K) molecules. This complex then recognizes the antioxidant responsive elements (ARE) in the promoter region of several genes, such as the cytoprotective heme oxygenase 1 (HMOX1), the phase II detoxification protein NAD(P)H quinine oxidoreductase (NQO1) and several genes involved in glutathione regulation. It is thought that skin sensitizers, which are known to be reactive to cysteine, are able to bind to the cysteine residues of Keap1 and thereby facilitate the release of Nrf2 (Motohashi & Yamamoto, 2004; Natsch, 2009). Although the majority of sensitizers can indeed bind to the cysteine residues, there are some that preferentially bind to lysine residues and these do not activate Nrf2 (Gerberick et al., 2007b; Natsch, 2009).

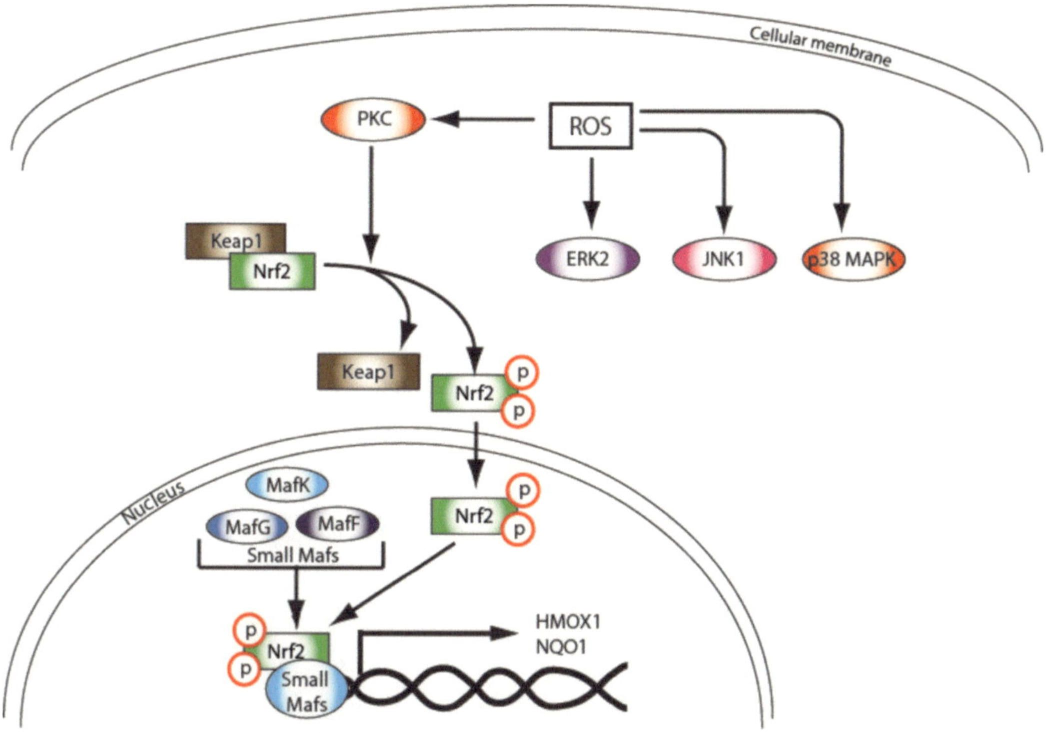

Fig. 3. The Nrf2-Keap1 pathway (adapted from biocarta, available at: http://www.biocarta.com/pathfiles/h_ARENRF2PATHWAY.asp)

It can be hypothesized that Nrf2 plays different roles in skin sensitization. First, Nrf2 activation is a result of oxidative stress induced by sensitizer exposure. Second, Nrf2 is involved in the regulation of the immune response, since several genes that are under Nrf2 control have been shown to have immunological effects. For example, upregulation of HMOX1 has been shown to inhibit the maturation of dendritic cells, thereby reducing T cell activation. Furthermore, HMOX1 induces an increased expression of the anti-inflammatory cytokine IL-10 (Listopad et al., 2007). Nrf2 has been shown to be important in attenuating different inflammatory responses (Kim et al., 2010). In Nrf2 deficient mice, the severity of disease in a colitis model was aggravated and this was attributed to increased levels of IL1-β, IL-6, IL12p40, and TNF-α, (Khor et al., 2006). In old mice deficient of Nrf2, skin sensitization was less pronounced, meaning that Nrf2 is essential for the skin sensitization process (Kim et al., 2008). Hence, Nrf2 has an important role in regulating immune responses.

Since skin sensitization involves different cell types, signaling pathways, cytokines and chemokines it might be possible that there is a direct link between Nrf2 activation and TLR activation. Nrf2 is involved in protection against oxidative stress and the induction of antioxidants. Activation of this pathway could affect redox-sensitive factors associated with TLR activation, such as NF-κB (Kim et al., 2010) and chemokines (Sozzani et al., 2005). For example, in cells exposed to LPS or nickel, the levels of thioredoxin-1 (Trx-1), an enzyme that is regulated by Nrf2, were elevated. It is postulated that the production of reactive oxygen species following TLR4 activation causes Nrf2 translocation and transcription of the target genes (Listopad et al., 2007; Rushworth et al., 2008). Evidence for a direct link between Nrf2 and TLR was found in *in vitro* studies in macrophages. It was shown that Nrf2 activation by LPS was dependent on MyD88 but independent of the production of reactive oxygen species, indicating a second induction mechanism for Nrf2. It was speculated that MyD88 dependent signaling induced via TLR4 leads to activation of Nrf2 in order to regulate the inflammatory response (Kim et al., 2011). It remains unclear if there is a link between Nrf2 and TLR activation in skin sensitization and more research is needed to better understand the underlying mechanisms of skin sensitization.

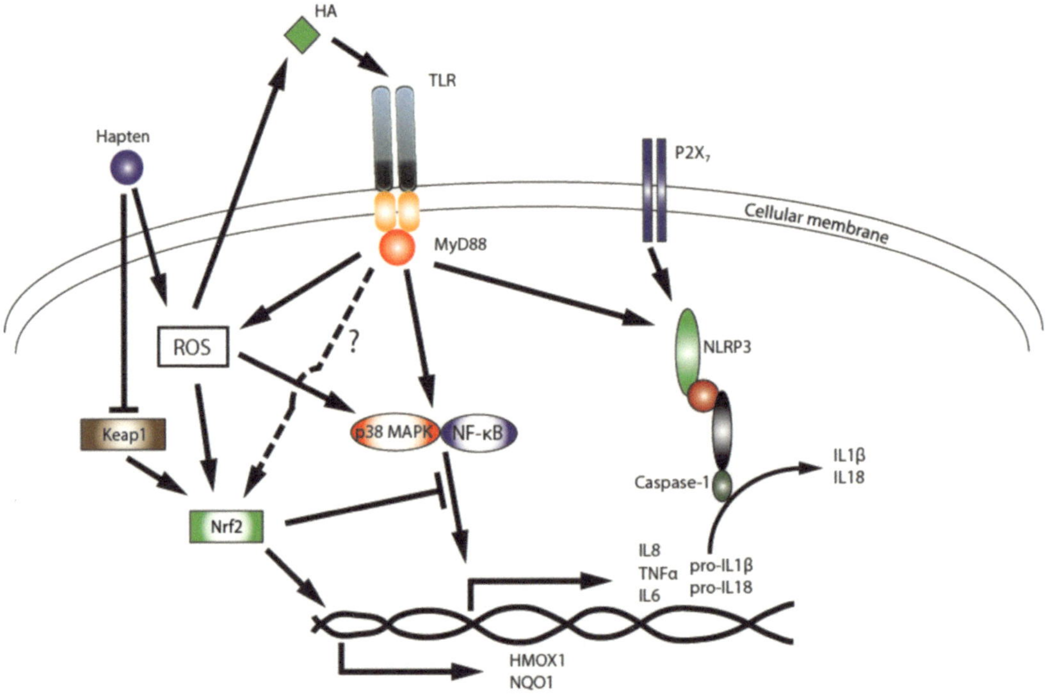

Fig. 4. Schematic overview of innate immune responses induced by sensitizers. Hapten exposure leads to degradation of hyaluronic acid (HA) in the skin and the HA fragments act as endogenous ligands for TLR activation. Downstream signaling pathways such as p38 MAPK are activated leading to NF-kB activation and release of pro-inflammatory cytokines (IL-6, IL-8, TNF-α) in the skin. At the same time, stress induced by haptens activates the NLRP3 inflammasome leading to caspase-1 activation and processing pro-IL-1β and pro-IL18 and subsequent release of IL-1β and IL-18. Together, this cascade of signaling pathways results in the essential factors needed for the development of an adaptive immune response to the skin sensitizers. On the other hand, the hapten exposure activates the Nrf2 pathway through generation of ROS and binding to Keap1, releasing Nrf2. Leading to production of antioxidants, affecting the redox balance. Redox-sensitive signaling pathways, such as p38 MAPK, NF-κB and chemokine production are attenuated in an attempt to reduce the inflammatory response in the skin and prevent skin sensitization (adapted from Martin et al., 2011).

5. Opportunities for the development of *in vitro* keratinocyte-based assays to predict the sensitizing potential of chemicals

In recent years many efforts have been made to develop cell-based assays able to identify skin sensitizers and to distinguish them from irritants. In keratinocyte-based assays, cytokine induction or gene expression profiles were assessed to find predictive biomarkers or pathways. In the human keratinocyte cell line HaCaT it was shown that intracellular IL-18 was significantly upregulated after exposure to four sensitizers and not after exposure to irritants (Van Och et al., 2005). Similarly, in the keratinocyte cell line NCTC2544 IL-18 was found to be predictive for skin sensitizers, and to distinguish them from respiratory sensitizers and irritants. Prohaptens require metabolic activation to become sensitizers were included in this assay and could be identified as well, indicating that these cells have sufficient metabolic activity (Corsini et al., 2009). IL-18 production is dependent on caspase-1 and requires the inflammasome activation. The relevance of signal transduction pathways in skin sensitizer induced IL-18 production was demonstrated using selective inhibitors and revealed a role for oxidative stress, NF-κB and p38 MAPK activation (Van Och et al., 2005; Corsini et al., 2009; Galbiati et al., 2011). In a reconstructed human epidermis model cytokine profiling was used to discriminate skin sensitizers from irritants. Five sensitizers and three irritants were tested in this 3D model and it was shown that sensitizers induce IL-8 production and secrete only low levels of IL-1α. In contrast, irritants induce high levels of IL-1α and only low levels of IL-8. With this limited number of substances the ratio of IL-8/ IL-1α could be used to distinguish sensitizers from irritants. The benefits of using a 3D skin model are the possibilities to test topical formulations and compounds with low water solubility (Coquette et al., 2003) .

Tools that can be used to identify biomarkers for specific toxic effects, such as skin sensitization, include "omics" technologies, such as transcriptomics (measuring mRNA expression) and proteomics (measuring protein expression in tissues or cells). Transcriptomics has been used in the HaCaT cell line to find genes that are able to distinguish between sensitizers and irritants. After exposure to eight sensitizers and six irritants, pathway analysis showed that the Nrf2 pathway was significantly affected by sensitizers while it was not triggered by irritants. In addition, a set of 13 genes was identified that could predict the sensitizing potential of chemicals with 73% accuracy (Vandebriel et al., 2010). Further research is needed to confirm the accuracy of this gene list when more substances are used. The relevance of Nrf2 for skin sensitization was confirmed using primary keratinocytes exposed to two skin sensitizers (Yoshikawa et al., 2010)

The importance of Nrf2 in skin sensitization has resulted in the development of a reporter cell line from the HaCaT cell line, the KeratinoSens assay (Natsch, 2009). The promoter sequence of the Nrf2 dependent human gene AKR1C2, coding for an aldo-keto reductase, was placed before the gene encoding luciferase. The principle of this assay is that exposure to skin sensitizers leads to activation of the Nrf2 pathway and luciferase expression. In this assay, 67 substances (sensitizers, non-sensitizers and irritants) were tested. A fold increase of 1.5 in luciferase expression was used to identify skin sensitizers and it was shown that accuracy of this assay was 85.1% (Natsch, 2009; Emter et al., 2010). In a ring study with five laboratories it was shown that the KeratinoSens assay was easy transferable to other laboratories. The accuracy of the assay was tested with 28 blinded test compounds and the assay was reproducible between the laboratories (Natsch et al., 2011).

The limitation of these keratinocyte based *in vitro* assays is that they only provide a yes/no answer and are currently not able to predict the potency of compounds. For classification and labeling purposes, it is essential to have a test method that can predict both the potential and potency of skin sensitizing chemicals. Sensitizing potency has been assessed in an assay using an *in vitro* reconstructed human epidermal equivalent. This model has been developed to determine the potency of skin irritants (Spiekstra et al., 2009). To asses if this model could be used for skin sensitizing potency as well, viability and IL-1α secretion were assessed after 24 hour of exposure to 12 substances. It was shown that potency estimates could be derived, but only for sensitizers with irritant and cytotoxic properties. Furthermore, the endpoints chosen were not able to distinguish between sensitizers and irritants. It has been proposed that this 3D skin model could be used in a tiered approach where it is combined with an assay capable of making this distinction, for example measuring IL-18 in the NCTC2544 cell line. More substances need to be tested in order to establish if potency estimates can be made for skin sensitizers (dos Santos et al., 2011). Furthermore, in the development of *in vitro* tests more attention should be given to this by focusing on dose-response relations and establish if these correlate to human and LLNA potency values.

Keratinocyte-based *in vitro* assays appear to be promising for the identification of skin sensitizers, but represent only one aspect of the skin sensitization process. However, it is not foreseen that hazard identification can be accomplished with one single test, but that a battery approach combining several alternative test methods should be used. In such an integrated testing strategy (ITS), other alternative skin sensitization tests that could be included are *in silico* approaches, such as quantitative structure activity relationship (QSAR) models. Characteristic physical-chemical properties of skin sensitizers, such as electrophilic reactivity and hydrophobicity, can be assessed in this approach. The reaction mechanisms for skin sensitizers have been defined in five applicability domains (Roberts et al., 2008). A promising assay for evaluation of the protein binding capacity *in chemico* is the Direct Peptide Binding Reactivity Assay (DPRA), in which the binding of substances to synthetic peptides is measured by HPLC analysis. The accuracy of this assay is 89% and this assay is currently in prevalidation at the European Centre for the Validation of Alternative Methods (ECVAM) (Gerberick et al., 2007b; Gerberick et al., 2009). Besides keratinocyte based assays, *in vitro* assays using dendritic cells could be included in an ITS. The activation and maturation of dendritic cells can be analyzed using several assays, such as the Myeloid U937 skin sensitization test (MUSST) and the human cell line activation test (h-CLAT). Both assays apply chemicals to a monocytic cell line, U937 and THP-1 respectively, and measure the upregulation of CD86 protein on the cell surface. In addition to CD86, the upregulation of CD54 is measured in the h-CLAT assay (Sakaguchi et al., 2006; Sakaguchi et al., 2007; Sakaguchi et al., 2009; Ashikaga et al., 2010). Both assays are currently in ECVAM prevalidation. Finally, T cell proliferation induced by chemical exposure is important to demonstrate if a substance is immunogenic and is comparable to the endpoint measured in the LLNA. T cell activation is evaluated by first exposing dendritic cells to chemicals; the dendritic cells will load their MHC with haptenized peptides and upregulate costimulatory molecules. Next, these chemical-exposed activated dendritic cells are added to autologous peripheral blood mononuclear cells (PBMC) from which immune regulatory cells have been removed. Naïve T cells that are able to recognize the hapten are activated and start to proliferate (Martin et al., 2010). The sensitivity of this assay has not been shown to date and this should be further explored.

Much progress is currently being made in the development of alternative (non-animal) test methods. However, it is as yet unclear how these different tests could be best combined in an ITS approach in order to make an accurate prediction of skin sensitizing potential and even more challenging: potency. An important step towards an ITS will be the development of a database in which all current outcomes per chemical and assay are listed in a matrix. In this database LLNA (or GPMT) data and human data should be included as well. This will allow evaluation of the sensitivity and specificity of a specific assay. In addition, such an approach can be applied to study the relationship between the various alternative assays and to get insight in the applicability domain of the individual assays. Another aspect is the relative importance of each assay for the outcome of the ITS. This will improve hazard identification as well as identify the key step(s) in the sensitization process (Vandebriel & van Loveren, 2010). In the integration of the results predefined weight factors for each assay should be summed and this sum is then used for prediction of skin sensitizing potential (Jowsey et al., 2006). To date, the applicability of ITS in this area has not been studied extensively. Natsch et al. (2009) integrated data of 116 chemicals from different *in vitro* and *in silico* assays. They used (1) peptide reactivity, (2) ARE induction in the KeratinoSens® assay, (3) calculated octanol-water partition coefficient (LogP) and (4) *in silico* TImes MEtabolism Simulator platform used for predicting Skin Sensitization (TIMES-SS), and compared the outcomes to LLNA data. It was shown that peptide reactivity and ARE induction similarly contributed to the model, whereas log*P* had only negligible contribution (TIMES-SS was not included in this analysis). The prediction accuracy for the optimized ITS model was 87.9% (Natsch et al., 2009). In an interlaboratory validation of four assays tested with 23 chemicals it was shown that the accuracy of the individual assays (DPRA, MUSST, h-CLAT and KeratinoSens®) ranged from 83-91%. However, the accuracy increased when the different assays were combined and the combination of KeratinoSens® with the MUSST resulted in 100% accuracy for these 23 chemicals (Bauch et al., 2011). Although these data are promising, the way in which the individual assays were combined should be clarified, since this was not well described in the paper. This approach should therefore be further validated with additional chemicals and a predefined ITS approach.

In the future the safety evaluation of skin sensitizers might be possible without using animal tests. Current hurdles are the need for alternative test systems that can also provide potency estimates. Also, the concept of ITS should be further developed with a focus on formulating guidelines on which assays should be included in a strategy. The most logical way forward is that of a weight of evidence approach. In a recent expert meeting arranged by the EU, it was foreseen that replacement of the current animal test for the hazard identification skin sensitization would take at least 5 to 7 years, but that it is unknown when a more quantitative approach is possible without experimental animals (Adler et al., 2011).

6. Acknowledgements

We acknowledge Lya Hernandez and Martijn Dollé from the National Institute for Public Health and the Environment for critically reading this chapter. Part of this work was funded by the Netherlands Genomics Initiative Organization for Scientific Research (NWO): nr. 050-060-510.

7. References

Ade N, Leon F, Pallardy M, Peiffer JL, Kerdine-Romer S, Tissier MH, Bonnet PA, Fabre I & Ourlin JC (2009) HMOX1 and NQO1 genes are upregulated in response to contact sensitizers in dendritic cells and THP-1 cell line: role of the Keap1/Nrf2 pathway. *Toxicol Sci* 107, 451-460.

Adler S, Basketter D, Creton S, Pelkonen O, van Benthem J, Zuang V, Andersen KE, Angers-Loustau A, Aptula A, Bal-Price A, Benfenati E, Bernauer U, Bessems J, Bois FY, Boobis A, Brandon E, Bremer S, Broschard T, Casati S, Coecke S, Corvi R, Cronin M, Daston G, Dekant W, Felter S, Grignard E, Gundert-Remy U, Heinonen T, Kimber I, Kleinjans J, Komulainen H, Kreiling R, Kreysa J, Leite SB, Loizou G, Maxwell G, Mazzatorta P, Munn S, Pfuhler S, Phrakonkham P, Piersma A, Poth A, Prieto P, Repetto G, Rogiers V, Schoeters G, Schwarz M, Serafimova R, Tahti H, Testai E, van Delft J, van Loveren H, Vinken M, Worth A & Zaldivar JM (2011) Alternative (non-animal) methods for cosmetics testing: current status and future prospects-2010. *Arch Toxicol* 85, 367-485.

Akiba H, Satoh M, Iwatsuki K, Kaiserlian D, Nicolas JF & Kaneko F (2004) CpG immunostimulatory sequences enhance contact hypersensitivity responses in mice. *J Invest Dermatol* 123, 488-493.

Albanesi C (2010) Keratinocytes in allergic skin diseases. *Curr Opin Allergy Clin Immunol* 10, 452-456.

Albanesi C, Scarponi C, Giustizieri ML & Girolomoni G (2005) Keratinocytes in inflammatory skin diseases. *Curr Drug Targets Inflamm Allergy* 4, 329-334.

Antonios D, Ade N, Kerdine-Römer S, Assaf-Vandecasteele H, Larangé A, Azouri H & Pallardy M (2009) Metallic haptens induce differential phenotype of human dendritic cells through activation of mitogen-activated protein kinase and NF-[kappa]B pathways. *Toxicology in Vitro* 23, 227-234.

Antonios D, Rousseau P, Larangé A, Kerdine-Römer S & Pallardy M (2010) Mechanisms of IL-12 Synthesis by Human Dendritic Cells Treated with the Chemical Sensitizer NiSO4. *The Journal of Immunology* 185, 89-98.

Antonopoulos C, Cumberbatch M, Dearman RJ, Daniel RJ, Kimber I & Groves RW (2001) Functional caspase-1 is required for Langerhans cell migration and optimal contact sensitization in mice. *J Immunol* 166, 3672-3677.

Ashikaga T, Sakaguchi H, Sono S, Kosaka N, Ishikawa M, Nukada Y, Miyazawa M, Ito Y, Nishiyama N & Itagaki H (2010) A comparative evaluation of in vitro skin sensitisation tests: the human cell-line activation test (h-CLAT) versus the local lymph node assay (LLNA). *Altern Lab Anim* 38, 275-284.

Bauch C, Kolle SN, Fabian E, Pachel C, Ramirez T, Wiench B, Wruck CJ, Ravenzwaay BV & Landsiedel R (2011) Intralaboratory validation of four in vitro assays for the prediction of the skin sensitizing potential of chemicals. *Toxicol In Vitro.*

Berard F, Marty JP & Nicolas JF (2003) Allergen penetration through the skin. *Eur J Dermatol* 13, 324-330.

Boehme KW & Compton T (2004) Innate sensing of viruses by toll-like receptors. *J Virol* 78, 7867-7873.

Coquette A, Berna N, Vandenbosch A, Rosdy M, De Wever B & Poumay Y (2003) Analysis of interleukin-1alpha (IL-1alpha) and interleukin-8 (IL-8) expression and release in in vitro reconstructed human epidermis for the prediction of in vivo skin irritation and/or sensitization. *Toxicol In Vitro* 17, 311-321.

Corsini E, Mitjans M, Galbiati V, Lucchi L, Galli CL & Marinovich M (2009) Use of IL-18 production in a human keratinocyte cell line to discriminate contact sensitizers from irritants and low molecular weight respiratory allergens. *Toxicol In Vitro* 23, 789-796.

Cumberbatch M, Dearman RJ, Antonopoulos C, Groves RW & Kimber I (2001) Interleukin (IL)-18 induces Langerhans cell migration by a tumour necrosis factor-alpha- and IL-1beta-dependent mechanism. *Immunology* 102, 323-330.

dos Santos GG, Spiekstra SW, Sampat-Sardjoepersad SC, Reinders J, Scheper RJ & Gibbs S (2011) A potential in vitro epidermal equivalent assay to determine sensitizer potency. *Toxicol In Vitro* 25, 347-357.

Feldmeyer L, Werner S, French LE & Beer HD (2010) Interleukin-1, inflammasomes and the skin. *Eur J Cell Biol* 89, 638-644.

Freudenberg MA, Esser PR, Jakob T, Galanos C & Martin SF (2009) Innate and adaptive immune responses in contact dermatitis: analogy with infections. *G Ital Dermatol Venereol* 144, 173-185.

Galbiati V, Mitjans M, Lucchi L, Viviani B, Galli CL, Marinovich M & Corsini E (2011) Further development of the NCTC 2544 IL-18 assay to identify in vitro contact allergens. *Toxicol In Vitro* 25, 724-732.

Gaspari AA (1997) The role of keratinocytes in the phatophysiology of contact dermatitis. *Contact Dermatitis* 17, 377-405.

Gelardi A, Morini F, Dusatti F, Penco S & Ferro M (2001) Induction by xenobiotics of phase I and phase II enzyme activities in the human keratinocyte cell line NCTC 2544. *Toxicol In Vitro* 15, 701-711.

Gerberick GF, Ryan CA, Dearman RJ & Kimber I (2007a) Local lymph node assay (LLNA) for detection of sensitization capacity of chemicals. *Methods* 41, 54-60.

Gerberick GF, Troutman JA, Foertsch LM, Vassallo JD, Quijano M, Dobson RL, Goebel C & Lepoittevin JP (2009) Investigation of peptide reactivity of pro-hapten skin sensitizers using a peroxidase-peroxide oxidation system. *Toxicol Sci* 112, 164-174.

Gerberick GF, Vassallo JD, Foertsch LM, Price BB, Chaney JG & Lepoittevin JP (2007b) Quantification of chemical peptide reactivity for screening contact allergens: a classification tree model approach. *Toxicol Sci* 97, 417-427.

Gunzer M, Riemann H, Basoglu Y, Hillmer A, Weishaupt C, Balkow S, Benninghoff B, Ernst B, Steinert M, Scholzen T, Sunderkotter C & Grabbe S (2005) Systemic administration of a TLR7 ligand leads to transient immune incompetence due to peripheral-blood leukocyte depletion. *Blood* 106, 2424-2432.

Hosogi M, Tonogaito H, Aioi A, Hamada K, Shimoda K, Muromoto R, Matsuda T & Miyachi Y (2004) Hapten-induced contact hypersensitivity is enhanced in Tyk2-deficient mice. *J Dermatol Sci* 36, 51-56.

Jin H, Kumar L, Mathias C, Zurakowski D, Oettgen H, Gorelik L & Geha R (2009) Toll-like receptor 2 is important for the T(H)1 response to cutaneous sensitization. *J Allergy Clin Immunol* 123, 875-882 e871.

Jowsey IR, Basketter DA, Westmoreland C & Kimber I (2006) A future approach to measuring relative skin sensitising potency: a proposal. *J Appl Toxicol* 26, 341-350.

Kawai T & Akira S (2009) The roles of TLRs, RLRs and NLRs in pathogen recognition. *Int Immunol* 21, 317-337.

Kawai T & Akira S (2010) The role of pattern-recognition receptors in innate immunity: update on Toll-like receptors. *Nat Immunol* 11, 373-384.

Khor TO, Huang M-T, Kwon KH, Chan JY, Reddy BS & Kong A-N (2006) Nrf2-Deficient Mice Have an Increased Susceptibility to Dextran Sulfate Sodium–Induced Colitis. *Cancer Research* 66, 11580-11584.

Kim HJ, Barajas B, Wang M & Nel AE (2008) Nrf2 activation by sulforaphane restores the age-related decrease of T(H)1 immunity: role of dendritic cells. *J Allergy Clin Immunol* 121, 1255-1261 e1257.

Kim J, Cha YN & Surh YJ (2010) A protective role of nuclear factor-erythroid 2-related factor-2 (Nrf2) in inflammatory disorders. *Mutat Res* 690, 12-23.

Kim KH, Lyu JH, Koo ST, Oh SR, Lee HK, Ahn KS, Sadikot RT & Joo M (2011) MyD88 is a mediator for the activation of Nrf2. *Biochem Biophys Res Commun* 404, 46-51.

Kimber I, Basketter DA, Gerberick GF & Dearman RJ (2002a) Allergic contact dermatitis. *Int Immunopharmacol* 2, 201-211.

Kimber I, Cumberbatch M, Dearman RJ & Griffiths CE (2002b) Danger signals and skin sensitization. *Br J Dermatol* 147, 613-614.

Kimber I & Dearman RJ (2002) Allergic contact dermatitis: the cellular effectors. *Contact Dermatitis* 46, 1-5.

Kimber I, Dearman RJ, Scholes EW & Basketter DA (1994) The local lymph node assay: developments and applications. *Toxicology* 93, 13-31.

Klekotka PA, Yang L & Yokoyama WM (2010) Contrasting roles of the IL-1 and IL-18 receptors in MyD88-dependent contact hypersensitivity. *J Invest Dermatol* 130, 184-191.

Kollisch G, Kalali BN, Voelcker V, Wallich R, Behrendt H, Ring J, Bauer S, Jakob T, Mempel M & Ollert M (2005) Various members of the Toll-like receptor family contribute to the innate immune response of human epidermal keratinocytes. *Immunology* 114, 531-541.

Kumar H, Kawai T & Akira S (2009) Pathogen recognition in the innate immune response. *Biochem J* 420, 1-16.

Latz E (2010) The inflammasomes: mechanisms of activation and function. *Curr Opin Immunol* 22, 28-33.

Lebre MC, van der Aar AM, van Baarsen L, van Capel TM, Schuitemaker JH, Kapsenberg ML & de Jong EC (2007) Human keratinocytes express functional Toll-like receptor 3, 4, 5, and 9. *J Invest Dermatol* 127, 331-341.

Listopad J, Asadullah K, Sievers C, Ritter T, Meisel C, Sabat R & Docke WD (2007) Heme oxygenase-1 inhibits T cell-dependent skin inflammation and differentiation and function of antigen-presenting cells. *Exp Dermatol* 16, 661-670.

Liu L, Inoue H, Nakayama H, Kanno R & Kanno M (2007) The endogenous danger signal uric Acid augments contact hypersensitivity responses in mice. *Pathobiology* 74, 177-185.

Martin SF, Dudda JC, Bachtanian E, Lembo A, Liller S, Durr C, Heimesaat MM, Bereswill S, Fejer G, Vassileva R, Jakob T, Freudenberg N, Termeer CC, Johner C, Galanos C & Freudenberg MA (2008) Toll-like receptor and IL-12 signaling control susceptibility to contact hypersensitivity. *J Exp Med* 205, 2151-2162.

Martin SF, Esser PR, Schmucker S, Dietz L, Naisbitt DJ, Park BK, Vocanson M, Nicolas JF, Keller M, Pichler WJ, Peiser M, Luch A, Wanner R, Maggi E, Cavani A, Rustemeyer T, Richter A, Thierse HJ & Sallusto F (2010) T-cell recognition of chemicals, protein allergens and drugs: towards the development of in vitro assays. *Cell Mol Life Sci* 67, 4171-4184.

Martin SF, Esser PR, Weber FC, Jakob T, Freudenberg MA, Schmidt M & Goebeler M (2011) Mechanisms of chemical-induced innate immunity in allergic contact dermatitis. *Allergy*.

Matos TJ, Duarte CB, Gonçalo M & Lopes MC (2005) DNFB activates MAPKs and upregulates CD40 in skin-derived dendritic cells. *Journal of Dermatological Science* 39, 113-123.

Matsue H, Edelbaum D, Shalhevet D, Mizumoto N, Yang C, Mummert ME, Oeda J, Masayasu H & Takashima A (2003) Generation and function of reactive oxygen species in dendritic cells during antigen presentation. *J Immunol* 171, 3010-3018.

Mehrotra P, Mishra KP, Raman G & Banerjee G (2005) Differential regulation of free radicals (reactive oxygen and nitrogen species) by contact allergens and irritants in human keratinocyte cell line. *Toxicol Mech Methods* 15, 343-350.

Mehrotra P, Upadhyaya S, Sinkar VP, Banerjee G & Mishra KP (2007) Differential phosphorylation of MAPK isoforms in keratinocyte cell line by contact allergens and irritant. *Toxicol Mech Methods* 17, 101-107.

Metz M & Maurer M (2009) Innate immunity and allergy in the skin. *Curr Opin Immunol* 21, 687-693.

Mitjans M, Galbiati V, Lucchi L, Viviani B, Marinovich M, Galli CL & Corsini E (2010) Use of IL-8 release and p38 MAPK activation in THP-1 cells to identify allergens and to assess their potency in vitro. *Toxicol In Vitro* 24, 1803-1809.

Miyazawa M, Ito Y, Kosaka N, Nukada Y, Sakaguchi H, Suzuki H & Nishiyama N (2008) Role of MAPK signaling pathway in the activation of dendritic type cell line, THP-1, induced by DNCB and NiSO4. *J Toxicol Sci* 33, 51-59.

Motohashi H & Yamamoto M (2004) Nrf2-Keap1 defines a physiologically important stress response mechanism. *Trends Mol Med* 10, 549-557.

Nakae S, Naruse-Nakajima C, Sudo K, Horai R, Asano M & Iwakura Y (2001) IL-1 alpha, but not IL-1 beta, is required for contact-allergen-specific T cell activation during the sensitization phase in contact hypersensitivity. *Int Immunol* 13, 1471-1478.

Natsch A (2009) The Nrf2-Keap1-ARE toxicity pathway as a cellular sensor for skin sensitizers -functional relevance and a hypothesis on innate reactions to skin sensitizers. *Toxicol Sci*.

Natsch A, Bauch C, Foertsch LM, Gerberick GF, Norman K, Hilberer A, Inglis H, Landsiedel R, Onken S, Reuter H, Schepky A & Emter R (2011) The intra- and inter-laboratory reproducibility and predictivity of the KeratinoSens assay to predict skin sensitizers in vitro: Results of a ring-study in five laboratories. *Toxicology in Vitro* 25, 733-744.

Natsch A, Emter R & Ellis G (2009) Filling the concept with data: integrating data from different in vitro and in silico assays on skin sensitizers to explore the battery approach for animal-free skin sensitization testing. *Toxicol Sci* 107, 106-121.

Nestle FO, Di Meglio P, Qin JZ & Nickoloff BJ (2009) Skin immune sentinels in health and disease. *Nat Rev Immunol* 9, 679-691.

Niture SK, Jain AK & Jaiswal AK (2009) Antioxidant-induced modification of INrf2 cysteine 151 and PKC-delta-mediated phosphorylation of Nrf2 serine 40 are both required for stabilization and nuclear translocation of Nrf2 and increased drug resistance. *J Cell Sci* 122, 4452-4464.

Novak N, Baurecht H, Schafer T, Rodriguez E, Wagenpfeil S, Klopp N, Heinrich J, Behrendt H, Ring J, Wichmann E, Illig T & Weidinger S (2008) Loss-of-function mutations in the filaggrin gene and allergic contact sensitization to nickel. *J Invest Dermatol* 128, 1430-1435.

Olaru F & Jensen LE (2010) Chemokine expression by human keratinocyte cell lines after activation of Toll-like receptors. *Exp Dermatol* 19, e314-316.

Python F, Goebel C & Aeby P (2009) Comparative DNA microarray analysis of human monocyte derived dendritic cells and MUTZ-3 cells exposed to the moderate skin sensitizer cinnamaldehyde. *Toxicol Appl Pharmacol* 239, 273-283.

Roberts DW, Aptula AO, Patlewicz G & Pease C (2008) Chemical reactivity indices and mechanism-based read-across for non-animal based assessment of skin sensitisation potential. *Journal of Applied Toxicology* 28, 443-454.

Rushworth SA, MacEwan DJ & O'Connell MA (2008) Lipopolysaccharide-induced expression of NAD(P)H:quinone oxidoreductase 1 and heme oxygenase-1 protects against excessive inflammatory responses in human monocytes. *J Immunol* 181, 6730-6737.

Sakaguchi H, Ashikaga T, Miyazawa M, Kosaka N, Ito Y, Yoneyama K, Sono S, Itagaki H, Toyoda H & Suzuki H (2009) The relationship between CD86/CD54 expression and THP-1 cell viability in an in vitro skin sensitization test--human cell line activation test (h-CLAT). *Cell Biol Toxicol* 25, 109-126.

Sakaguchi H, Ashikaga T, Miyazawa M, Yoshida Y, Ito Y, Yoneyama K, Hirota M, Itagaki H, Toyoda H & Suzuki H (2006) Development of an in vitro skin sensitization test using human cell lines; human Cell Line Activation Test (h-CLAT). II. An inter-laboratory study of the h-CLAT. *Toxicol In Vitro* 20, 774-784.

Sakaguchi H, Miyazawa M, Yoshida Y, Ito Y & Suzuki H (2007) Prediction of preservative sensitization potential using surface marker CD86 and/or CD54 expression on human cell line, THP-1. *Arch Dermatol Res* 298, 427-437.

Schmidt M, Raghavan B, Muller V, Vogl T, Fejer G, Tchaptchet S, Keck S, Kalis C, Nielsen PJ, Galanos C, Roth J, Skerra A, Martin SF, Freudenberg MA & Goebeler M (2010) Crucial role for human Toll-like receptor 4 in the development of contact allergy to nickel. *Nat Immunol* 11, 814-819.

Seong SY & Matzinger P (2004) Hydrophobicity: an ancient damage-associated molecular pattern that initiates innate immune responses. *Nat Rev Immunol* 4, 469-478.

Son Y, Ito T, Ozaki Y, Tanijiri T, Yokoi T, Nakamura K, Takebayashi M, Amakawa R & Fukuhara S (2006) Prostaglandin E2 is a negative regulator on human plasmacytoid dendritic cells. *Immunology* 119, 36-42.

Sozzani S, Bosisio D, Mantovani A & Ghezzi P (2005) Linking stress, oxidation and the chemokine system. *Eur J Immunol* 35, 3095-3098.

Spiekstra SW, Dos Santos GG, Scheper RJ & Gibbs S (2009) Potential method to determine irritant potency in vitro - Comparison of two reconstructed epidermal culture models with different barrier competency. *Toxicol In Vitro* 23, 349-355.

Stutz A, Golenbock DT & Latz E (2009) Inflammasomes: too big to miss. *J Clin Invest* 119, 3502-3511.

Takanami-Ohnishi Y, Amano S, Kimura S, Asada S, Utani A, Maruyama M, Osada H, Tsunoda H, Irukayama-Tomobe Y, Goto K, Karin M, Sudo T & Kasuya Y (2002) Essential role of p38 mitogen-activated protein kinase in contact hypersensitivity. *J Biol Chem* 277, 37896-37903.

Trinchieri G & Sher A (2007) Cooperation of Toll-like receptor signals in innate immune defence. *Nat Rev Immunol* 7, 179-190.

Van Och FM, Van Loveren H, Van Wolfswinkel JC, Machielsen AJ & Vandebriel RJ (2005) Assessment of potency of allergenic activity of low molecular weight compounds based on IL-1alpha and IL-18 production by a murine and human keratinocyte cell line. *Toxicology* 210, 95-109.

Van Pelt FN, Meierink YJ, Blaauboer BJ & Weterings PJ (1990) Immunohistochemical detection of cytochrome P450 isoenzymes in cultured human epidermal cells. *J Histochem Cytochem* 38, 1847-1851.

Vandebriel RJ, Pennings JL, Baken KA, Pronk TE, Boorsma A, Gottschalk R & Van Loveren H (2010) Keratinocyte gene expression profiles discriminate sensitizing and irritating compounds. *Toxicol Sci* 117, 81-89.

Vandebriel RJ & van Loveren H (2010) Non-animal sensitization testing: state-of-the-art. *Crit Rev Toxicol* 40, 389-404.

Vocanson M, Hennino A, Rozieres A, Poyet G & Nicolas JF (2009) Effector and regulatory mechanisms in allergic contact dermatitis. *Allergy* 64, 1699-1714.

Weber FC, Esser PR, Muller T, Ganesan J, Pellegatti P, Simon MM, Zeiser R, Idzko M, Jakob T & Martin SF (2010) Lack of the purinergic receptor P2X(7) results in resistance to contact hypersensitivity. *J Exp Med* 207, 2609-2619.

Wheeler DS, Chase MA, Senft AP, Poynter SE, Wong HR & Page K (2009) Extracellular Hsp72, an endogenous DAMP, is released by virally infected airway epithelial cells and activates neutrophils via Toll-like receptor (TLR)-4. *Respir Res* 10, 31.

Yokoi S, Niizeki H, Iida H, Asada H & Miyagawa S (2009) Adjuvant effect of lipopolysaccharide on the induction of contact hypersensitivity to haptens in mice. *J Dermatol Sci* 53, 120-128.

Yoshikawa Y, Sasahara Y, Kitano Y, Kanazawa N, Shima H & Hashimoto-Tamaoki T (2010) Upregulation of genes orchestrating keratinocyte differentiation, including the novel marker gene ID2, by contact sensitizers in human bulge-derived keratinocytes. *J Biochem Mol Toxicol* 24, 10-20.

Yusuf N, Nasti TH, Huang CM, Huber BS, Jaleel T, Lin HY, Xu H & Elmets CA (2009) Heat shock proteins HSP27 and HSP70 are present in the skin and are important mediators of allergic contact hypersensitivity. *J Immunol* 182, 675-683.

Zhao Y, Balato A, Fishelevich R, Chapoval A, Mann DL & Gaspari AA (2009) Th17/Tc17 infiltration and associated cytokine gene expression in elicitation phase of allergic contact dermatitis. *Br J Dermatol* 161, 1301-1306.

Part 3

Patch Testing

4

Topical Delivery of Haptens: Methods of Modulation of the Cutaneous Permeability to Increase the Diagnosis of Allergic Contact Dermatitis

M. Nino, G. Calabrò and P. Santoianni
Department of Dermatology, University Federico II of Naples, Italy

1. Introduction

To be effective an active drug or principle must cross the stratum corneum barrier; this process can be influenced to obtain better functional and therapeutical effects. In spite of the wide variety of the methods studied in order to improve the transdermal transfer to obtain systemic effects, the applicability is limited in this field. Attention to the epidermal barrier and penetration of active principles has been reported mostly in studies concerning dermocosmetics. Studies regarding methods of penetration are gaining experimental and clinical interest. Cutaneous bioavailability of most commercially available dermatological formulations is low. Increase of intradermal delivery can relate to chemical, biochemical, or physical manipulations. Chemical enhancers have been adopted to: (a) increase the diffusibility of the substance across the barrier, (b) increase product solubility in the vehicle, (c) improve the partition coefficient. Moreover, methods of interference with the biosynthesis of some lipids allow the modification of the structure of the barrier to increase the penetration. Recent development of these methods are here reported and underline the importance and role of vehicles and other factors that determine effects of partition and diffusion, crucial to absorption of high molecular weight haptens in allergic contact dermatitis.

The skin represents an important barrier of the penetration of exogenous substances into the body and, on the other hand, a potential avenue for the transport of functional active principles into the skin and/or the body. Several studies have shown the modalities through which these molecules cross the horny layer, which represents the most important limiting factor of the process of diffusion and penetration, and have discussed how to increase the penetration of pharmacologically active substances **[1-3]**. The stratum corneum has a very peculiar structure: the corneocytes (the *bricks*: about 85% of the mass of horny mass) and intercellular lipids (15%) are arranged in approximately 15-20 layers. It consists of about 70 % proteins, 15 % lipids, and only 15 % water. In the corneocytes contain keratin, filagrin, and demolition products **[4]**. The corneocyte lacks lipids, but is rich in proteins. The lipids are inside extracellular spaces, in a bilayer organization surrounding corneocytes. The very low permeability of the horny layer to hydrosoluble substances is because of this extracellular lipid matrix. Cutaneous penetration of hydrophilic substances is limited because of the convoluted and tortuous intercellular space and hydrophobicity of three lipidic constituents: ceramides, cholesterol, and free fatty acids that are present in the molar ratio: 1: 1: 1 (weight ratio: ceramides 50%, cholesterol 35-40%, free fatty acids 10-15%) **[5].** This ratio is critical: because the diminution of the concentration of one of these types of lipids alters the molar ratio functional to the normality of the barrier and modifies its integrity **[6].** The variations of this lamellar structure and/or its lipid composition are the structural and biochemical basis of permeability variations along with the thickness of the horny layer. The extracellular matrix forms also the so-called the 'horny layer reservoir' (some substances are partially retained in the corneous layer and are slowly released) **[7-8].** Various processes carried out serially or in parallel, are involved in cutaneous penetration of substances and these may cross the stratum corneum via an intercellular or a transcellular route. Moreover, entrance through pilosebaceous units and eccrine glands is possible. Many efforts to obtain therapeutic effects in tissues far from the skin have been made. We may have: topical administration, with a pharmacological effect limited to skin, with some unavoidable systemic absorption; loco-regional delivery, when the therapeutic effect is obtained in tissues more or less deeply beneath the skin (muscles, articulations, vessels, etc.) with limited systemic absorption; and transdermic delivery that aims to obtain, through application of preparations on the skin, pharmacologically active levels for the treatment of systemic diseases through skin vascular network or for the diagnosis of a suspected contact dermatitis.

1.1 Stratum corneum barrier and intradermal delivery

The penetration through the stratum corneum involves partition phenomena of applied molecules between lipophilic and hydrophilic compartments. For many substances the penetration takes place through an intercellular way, more than transcellular, diffusing around the keratinocytes.

Intercellular movement. The lipid lamellae (each one including 2 or 3 bilayers and made mainly of ceramides, cholesterol, and free fatty acids) are the intercellular structure of the horny layer, with the main role in barrier function. Most solute substances, non-polar or polar, penetrate across intercellular lipid avenues. The permeability of very polar solutes is constant and similar to the transport of ions (e.g. potassium ions). Lipophilic solute permeability increases according to specific lipophilic properties.

Transcellular movement. Stratum corneum intracellular components are essentially devoid of lipids and lack a functional lipid matrix around keratin and keratohyalin. This results in an almost impenetrability of corneocytes [**9**]. Degradation of the corneodesmosomes causes formation of a continuous lacunar dominio ("aqueous pore") allowing intercellular penetration; the lacunae formed are scattered and not continuous, and form as a result of occlusion, ionophoresis, and ultrasound waves. These may become larger and connect forming a net ("pore-way"). Various methods can induce this type of permeability increase : physical and chemical methods [**10**].

Transport through follicular and gland structures. Movement through hair follicles, pilosebaceous units, and eccrine glands is limited. The orifices of the pilosebaceous units represent about 10 percent of all skin delivery in areas where their density is high (face and scalp) and only 0.1 percent in areas where their density is low. This is a possible selective way for some drugs. Follicular penetration may be influenced by sebaceous secretion, which favors the absorption of substances soluble in lipids. The penetration through the pilosebaceous units is dependent upon the property of the substance and type of preparation.

2. Role of the vehicle and excipients and interaction with the active principles

A vehicle is defined by the type of preparation (cream, ointment, gel) and the excipients (water, paraffin, propilen glycol); the terms "vehicle" and "excipient" refer to different entities.

Vehicle and excipients deeply influence the velocity and magnitude of absorption and consequently the bioavailability and efficacy. The excipients of the vehicle modulate the effects of partition and diffusion in the stratum corneum.

A lipid preparation that promotes occlusion may enhance the penetration of the drug, but ointments and lipid preparations are not always more powerful than creams. Creams, gels and solutions may be formulated so as to obtain an effect equivalent to that of ointments. Topical corticosteroids of different classes of potency may show the same activity when formulated in different vehicles. A gel preparation of kellin, obtaining better penetration, has demonstrated important results in the treatment of vitiligo. Also transfollicular penetration is influenced by vehicle and excipients; better results are given by lipophilic and alcoholic vehicles. Relevant factors include dimension and charge of the molecules of the solute.

3. Pharmacokinetic parameters - Vehicle/ corneous layer partition

For the purpose of the study of the mechanisms of transport and the functions of the skin barrier, it can be considered as a membrane or a cluster of membranes (mathematical principles can be applied) **[11]**. On the whole, transport through the horny layer is mainly a molecular passive diffusion. The physico-chemical and structural properties of the substance determine the capacity of diffusion and penetration through the membrane: important determinants are solubility and diffusibility.

The diffusibility and the ability of a solute to penetrate through the barrier is influenced by several factors including the tortuosity of the intercellular route. This passive process of absorption follows Fick's law of diffusion: the velocity of absorption - flow - is proportional to the difference of concentration of the substance in relation to that within the barrier. It can finally be noted that the permeability coefficient relates flow and concentration, resulting from partition coefficient, diffusion coefficient, and length of diffusion route **[12-16]**.

4. Conditions that modify the barrier function

During hydration the greater part of the water is associated with intracellular keratin; the natural factor of hydration or natural moisturizing factor (NMF) absorbs a noticeable amount of water (10% of the weight of the corneocyte). Corneocytes swell and the barrier properties of the stratum corneum are deeply altered. In the intercellular space the small amount of water linked to polar groups by hydration does not alter the organization of lipids and does not reduce of permeability **[17]**. The effect of the hydration however has a discontinuous effect; the increase in permeability may be by ten times for some substances and very limited for others **[18]**. Occlusion partially hinders the loss of humidity of the skin, increasing the content of water of the horny layer. However the NMF level in the horny layer is almost zero. It seems therefore that there is a homeostatic mechanism that prevents hyperhydration of the skin **[9]**. Occlusion may increase the absorption by several times, especially for hydrophilic compounds. However, in some conditions it may promote the formation of a reservoir effect. The acidity of the cutaneous surface, controlling homeostasis and enzymatic activities, influences permeability **[19]**; the metabolic activity of the skin (enzymatic oxidoreductive processes) may modify the substances applied, influencing permeability and effects.

Absorption is also influenced by other skin properties that vary at different cutaneous anatomical sites. For instance, the absorption diminishes greatly as one moves from the palpebral skin to the plantar surfaces **[20]**.

Age influences skin absorption. Various biological activities are lower in the skin of the aged individual. Great variation is also noted for the premature infant and neonate, who have greater cutaneous permeability **[21]**. There are no experimental data confirming the validity of friction on transcutaneous absorption **[6]**. Alterations of the barrier induce modifications of TEWL **[9]**. In addition, the horny layer may be defined as a biosensor; alterations of external humidity regulate proteolysis of filaggrin, synthesis of lipids, DNA, and proteins within keratinocytes, which can lead also to inflammatory phenomena **[22]**.

The cutaneous bioavailability of most commercial dermatological formulations IS about 1-5% of applied dose **[23]**.

The active substances of topical formulations are generally absorbed in small quantities; only a reduced fraction passes from the vehicle into the stratum corneum. The greater part remains on the surface of the skin, subject to loss in several ways such as by sweating, chemical degradation, and removal. Future standards would therefore aim to make formulations not merely high in concentration, but pharmaceutically optimized to have an elevated (50-100%) bioavailability. On the other hand, one must consider the marked variations of the different cutaneous areas and skin conditions that make uncertain the therapeutic equivalence when compared with other ways of administration in clinical conditions **[24]**.

5. Methods of modulation of cutaneous permeability

When a substance is applied on the skin with a simple vehicle the therapeutic result can be unsatisfactory because of the insufficient concentration obtained in the application area **[25]**. In the last few years strategies have been developed in order to increase the efficacy of the vehicle **[26]**. They may be of chemical, biochemical or physical order.

5.1 Chemical enhancers

In order to increase the penetration the vehicle may be integrated with enhancers that by interacting with intercellular lipids improve the diffusion coefficient of the substance in the stratum corneum. Chemical enhancers may: a) increase the diffusibility of the substance inside the barrier, b) increase the solubility in the vehicle or both, or c) improve the partition coefficient.

These substances may frequently have a not specific action. Enhancers of this type, that are not widely used, are Azone, Dermac SR-38, and oleic acid [27]. In some cases, however, these have an irritating effect and must be carefully evaluated in the various preparations [28].

Excipients like ethanol, propylene-glycol, and dimethylsulfoxide (DMSO) may increase the diffusion by altering the organization of lipids of the horny layer [29]. The interference with the biosynthesis of some lipids may alter the structure of the barrier and increase the penetration. Methods have also been studied that interfere with secretion and organization of lipids (e.g., brefeldine, monetine, and cloroquine). In addition, enhancers that alter the supramolecolar organization of the bistratified lamellae (synthetic analogs of fats, inducing abnormalities of the organization of the membranes; complex precursors that can not be metabolized, etc.) have been studied. These methods produce an alteration of the critical molar ratio among ceramides, cholesterol, and fatty acids; if there is decrease or excess of one of these 3 key lipids, the lamellar organization cannot be maintained. There may be separation of the phases with more permeable interestitial spaces and formation of a new way of penetration [30].

The efficacy of the enhancers may be increased by inhibition of the metabolic reaction of repair once the alteration of the barrier has been obtained. This would involve inhibiting metabolic sequences that can rebuild and maintain the barrier function. Inhibitors of enzymes with relevant functions (e.g., lovastatin) or specific inhibitors of enzymes synthesizing ceramides or fatty acids induces alteration of the molar ratio of the three critical lipids and leads to discontinuity in the lamellar layer system [31]. Other enhancements may be obtained by modifying the polarity [32].

The number of drugs for which transdermic methods for systemic use has been possible is very small and restricted to lipophilic and low molecular weight substances (e.g. nicotinic acid, nitroglycerin, clonidine, steroid hormones, and scopolamine) [33].

5.2 Carrier vesicular systems

Liposome formulations can be very effective. However, they probably increase penetration only through the transappendigeal avenue [34]. Niosomes and transferosomes, formed by modified liposomes (phosphatidilcoline, sodium cholate, ethanol), are systems based on the ability of vesicles to cross the unaltered horny layer because of the osmotic gradient between external and internal layers of the barrier. These are "flexible" vesicles able to transport their contents through the intercellular tortuous route of the corneous layer.

5.3 Scratch-patch test

Although closed patch tests are the mainstay for the evaluation of allergic contact dermatitis, occasionally, even when appropriate concentrations of allergens are used and contact allergy is strongly suspected, positive reactions are not always obtained. As in the cases that will be described patch test with high molecular weight substances as heparin, or low molecular weight as acyclovir may give doubtful results in sensitized patients, possibly due to poor penetration of this substances through the epidermis. Scratch–patch testing, by compromising epidermal barrier function, enables enhanced penetration of substances into the skin [**35-37**]. The method is performed by causing mechanical injury to the epidermis with a sterile skin prick lancet in order to compromise the stratum corneum, which represents the most important barrier limiting hapten penetration. The test reactions are usually read after D2 and D3, when possible, also after D4 and D7. The method of grading a positive scratch–patch test is identical to that used for conventional patch testing with no differences. It can be used for many drugs: low molecular wheight molecules (e.g. *β*-blockers, antiviral drugs etc.) and also high molecular wheight molecules (e.g. heparin etc.):

5.3.1 *β*-blockers

Contact allergy to topical *β*-blockers is a well-recognized side-effect of glaucoma treatment [**38-41**]. Sensitization may be singly to agents such as timolol, befunolol, levobunolol, or, more rarely, to multiple *β*-blockers in a single patient.

A closed patch test, usually used in clinical practice for the diagnosis of allergic contact dermatitis, is often sufficient to show *β*-blockers contact allergy. However, there may be difficulties in obtaining positive patch tests to *β*-blockers, as showed in earlier reports [**42-43**]. Poor penetration through intact skin on the back, where patch testing is normally applied, may be a factor.

5.3.2 Antiviral drugs

Topical antiviral drugs are frequently used, but although repeated applications can lead to contact reactions **[44-45]**, adverse cutaneous reactions are not commonly observed. Allergic contact dermatitis caused by acyclovir is rare, with only 20 studies reported **[46-48].** Because of the doubtful reactions with antiviral, especially acyclovir, and in view of the suggestive clinical history, we recommend the scratch–patch test followed by repeated open application test (ROAT).

5.3.3 Heparin

Heparin is a sulfated glycosaminoglycan with anticoagulant properties. It is usually injected intravenously or subcutaneously but is also available for topical application. Cutaneous allergic reactions due to subcutaneously injected heparin have been reported **[49-50].**

We report a case of patch-test-negative allergic contact dermatitis, diagnosed by scratch patch testing, from a gel containing heparin. Allergic reaction to subcutaneously injected heparins is not a rare occurrence **[51-52]** but there are only a few reports of contact dermatitis from topical heparin **[53].**

In cases of suspected contact allergy, when conventional closed patch test shows negative or doubtful results, scratch–patch testing should be considered. We recommend, after performing scratch-patch test, to execute a ROAT to be sure the drug can be applied safely.

6. References

[1] Dermatological and Transdermal Formulations. New York: Marcel Dekker, Inc; 2002.2. Bronaugh RL, Maibach HI. Percutaneous Absorption: Drugs - Cosmetics - Mechanisms - Methodology (Drugs and the Pharmaceutical Sciences). Informa Healthcare; 4th Ed;2005.

[2] Smith EW, Maibach HI. Penetration percutaneous enhancers. UK: Taylor and Francis, 2nd Ed; 2006.

[3] Lampe MA, Burlingame AL, Whitney J, Williams ML, Brown BE, Roitman E. Human stratum corneum lipids: characterization and regional differences. J Lipid Res 1983;24:120-30.

[4] Elias PM, Menon GK. Structural and lipid biochemical correlates of the epidermal permeability barrier. Adv Lipid Res 1991;24:1-26.

[5] Elias PM, Tsai JC, Menon GK, editor. Skin barrier, percutaneous drug delivery and pharmacokinetics. Mosby: Dermatology; 2003. p 1235-52.

[6] Elias PM, Feingold KR, Menon JK. The stratum corneum, two compartments model and its functional implication. In: Basel, Karger Shroot B, Shaefer H, editors. Skin Pharmacokinetics 1987. p 1-9.

[7] Surber C, Davis AF. Bioavailability and Bioequivalence of Dermatological Formulations In: Kenneth AW, editor. Dermatological and Transdermal Formulations. New York: Marcel Dekker, Inc; 2002. p 401-498.

[8] Roberts MS, Cross SE, Pellett MA. Skin transport. In: Kenneth AW, editor. Dermatological and Transdermal FormulationsNew York: Marcel Dekker, Inc; 2002. p 89-195.

[9] Menon GK, Elias PM. Morphologic basis for a pore-pathway in mammalian stratum corneum. Skin Pharmacol 1997;10:235-46.

[10] Watkinson AC, Brain KR. Basic mathematical principles in skin permeation.: In: Kenneth AW, editor. Dermatological and Transdermal Formulations. New York: Marcel Dekker, Inc; 2002. p 61-88.

[11] Franz TJ. Kinetics of cutaneous drug penetration. Int J Dermatol 1983;22:499-505.

[12] Franz TJ. Pharmacokinetics and skin in: Skin barrier, percutaneous drug delivery and pharmacokinetics. In: Jean LB, Joseph LJ, editor. Mosby: Dermatology; 2003. p 1969-78

[13] Orecchia G, Sangalli ME, Gazzaniga A, et al. Topical photochemotherapy of vitiligo with a new khellin formulation: preliminary clinical results. J Dermatol Treat 1998;9:65-9.

[14] Roberts M, Cross SE, Pellett MA. Skin transport In: Kenneth AW, editor. Dermatological and Transdermal Formulations. New York: Marcel Dekker, Inc; 2002.

[15] Middleton JD. The mechanism of water binding in stratum corneum. Br J Dermatol 1968;80:437-50.

[16] Horii I, Nakajama Y, Obate Ml. Stratum corneum hydration and aminoacids contant in xerotic skin. Br J Dermatol Res 1989;121:588-64.

[17] Imokawa G, Kuno H, Kawai M. Stratum corneum lipids serve as bound-water modulator. J Invest Dermatol 1991;96:845-51.

[18] Mauro T, Hollerann WM, Grayson S, Gao WN, Man MQ, Kriehuber E, et al. Barrier recovery is impeded at neutal pH, independent of ionic effects: implications for extracellular lipid processing. Arch Dermatol Res 1998;290:215-22.

[19] Rougier A, Lotte C, Corcuff TP. Relationship between skin permeability and cornecyte size according to anatomic site, age and sex in man. J Soc Cosmet Chem 1988;39:15-21.

[20] Berardesca E, Maibach HI. Racial differences in skin pathophysiology. J Am Acad Dermatol 1996;34:667-72.

[21] Menon GK, Elias PM, Feingold KR. Integrity of the permeability barrier is crucial for manteinance of the epidermal calcium gradient. Br J Dermatol 1994;130:139-47.

[22] Surber C, Davis AF. Bioavailability and Bioequivalence of Dermatological Formulations. In: Kenneth AW, editor. Dermatological and Transdermal Formulations. New York: Marcel Dekker, Inc;2002..p401-498.

[23] Hauck WW. Bioequivalence studies of topical preparations: statistical considerations. Int J Dermatol 1992;31 (suppl. 1):29-33.

[24] Skelly JP, Shah VP, Maibach HI. FDA and AAPS report of workshop on principles and practices of in vitro percutaneous penetration studies: relevance to bioavailability and bioequivalence. Pharm Res 1987;4:265-71.

[25] Shah VP, Elkins J, Hanus J, Noorizadeh C, Skelly JP. In vitro release fo hydrocortisone from topical preparations and automated procedure. Pharm Res 1991;8:55-9.

[26] Davis AF, Gyurik RJ, Hadgraft J. Formulation strategies for modulating skin permeation In: Kenneth AW, editor. Dermatological and Transdermal Formulations. New York: Marcel Dekker, Inc;2002.

[27] Patil S, Singh P, Szolar-Platzer C, Maibach HI. Epidermal enzymes as penetration enhancers in transdermal drug delivery? J Pharm Sci 1996;85:249-52.

[28] Mitragotri S. Synergistic effects of enhancers for transdermal drug delivery. Pharm Res 2000; 17:1354-9.

[29] Tsai JC, Guy RH, Thornfeldt CR, Gao WN, Feingold KR, Elias PM. Metabolic approaches to enhance transdermal drug delivery. Effect of lipid synthesis inhibitors. J Pharm Sci 1996;85:643-8.

[30] Johnson ME, Mitragotri S, Patel A, Blankschtein D, Langer R. Synergistic effects of chemical enhancers and therapeutic ultrasounds on transdermal drug delivery. J Pharm Sci 1996;85:670-9.

[31] Choi EH, Lee SH, Ahn SK, Hwang SM. The pretreatment effect of chemical skin penetration enhancers in transdermal drug delivery. Skin Pharmacol Appl Skin Physiol 1999;12:326-35.

[32] Singh J, Maibach HI. Transdermal delivery and cutaneous reactions. In: Kenneth AW, editor. Dermatological and Transdermal Formulations. New York: Marcel Dekker, Inc;2002. 34. Korting HC, Stolz W, Schmid MH, Maierhofer G. Interaction of liposomes with human epidermis reconstructed in vitro. Br J Dermatol 1995;132:571-9.

[33] Jappe U, Uter W, Menezes de Pádua C A, Herbst R A, Schnuch A. Allergic contact dermatitis due to beta-blockers in eye drops: a retrospective analysis of multicentre surveillance data 1993–2004. Acta Derm Venereol 2006:86:509–514.

[34] Holdiness MR. Contact dermatitis to topical drugs for glaucoma. Am J Contact Dermat 2001:12:217–9.
[35] Nino M, Suppa F, Ayala F, Balato N. Allergic contact dermatitis due to the beta-blocker befunolol in eyedrops, with cross-sensitivity to carteolol. Contact Dermatitis 2001:44:369.
[36] Katoh N, Kanzaki T. Contact dermatitis due to befunolol hydrochloride eyedrops. Contact Dermatitis 1997:10:1113–6.
[37] Van der Meeren H L, Meurs P. Sensitization to levobunolol eyedrops. Contact Dermatitis 1993:28:41–2.
[38] Quiralte J, Florido F, Saenz de San Pedro B. Allergic contact dermatitis from carteolol and timolol in eyedrops. Contact Dermatitis 2000:42:245.
[39] Corazza M, Virgili A, Mantovani L, Taddei Masieri L. Allergic contact dermatitis from cross-reacting β-blocking agents. Contact Dermatitis 1993:28:188–9.
[40] O'Donnell B F, Foulds I S. Contact allergy to beta-blocking agents in ophthalmic preparations. Contact Dermatitis 1993:28:121–2.
[41] Sánchez-Pérez J, Jesús Del Río M, Fernández-Villalta M J, García-Díez A. Positive use test in contact dermatitis from betaxolol hydrochloride. Contact Dermatitis 2002:46:313–4.
[42] Nino M, Balato N, Di Costanzo L, Gaudiello F. Scratch-patch test for the diagnosis of allergic contact dermatitis to aciclovir. Contact Dermatitis 2009:60:56–7.
[43] Serpentier-Daude A, Colet E, Didier A F et al. Contact dermatitis to topical antiviral drugs. Ann Dermatol Venereol 2000:127:191–4.
[44] Holdiness M R. Contact dermatitis from topical antiviral drugs. Contact Dermatitis 2001:44:265–9.
[45] Goh C. Compound allergy to Spectraban 15 lotion and Zovirax cream. Contact Dermatitis 1990:22:61–2.
[46] Vernassiere C, Barbaud A, Trechot P H et al. Systemic acyclovir reaction subsequent to acyclovir contact allergy: which systemic antiviral drug should then be used? Contact Dermatitis 2003:49:155–7.
[47] Lammintausta K, Makela L, Kalimo K. Rapid systemic valaciclovir reaction subsequent to aciclovir contact allergy. Contact Dermatitis 2001:45:181.
[48] Maroto-Iitani M, Higaki Y, Kawashima M. Cutaneous allergic reaction to heparins: subcutaneous but not intravenous provocation Contact Dermatitis 2005;52:228–30.
[49] Hohenstein E, Tsakiris D, Bircher AJ. Delayed-type hypersensitivity to the ultra-low-molecular-weight heparin fondaparinux. Contact Dermatitis 2004;51:149-51.
[50] Jappe U, Juschka U, Kuner N, Hausen BM, Krohn K.. Fondaparinux: a suitable alternative in cases of delayed-type allergy to heparins and semisynthetic heparinoids? A study of 7 cases. Contact Dermatitis 2004;51:67–72.
[51] Schindewolf M, Ludwig RJ, Wolter M, Himsel A, Zgouras D, Kaufmann R, et al. Tolerance of fondaparinux in patients with generalized contact dermatitis to heparin. J Eur Acad Dermatol Venereol 2008;22:378–80.

[52] Nino M, Patruno C, Zagaria O, Balato N. Allergic contact dermatitis from heparin-containing gel: use of scratch patch test for diagnosis. Dermatitis 2009: 20: 171–172.

5

Progress on the Development of Human *In Vitro* Assays for Assessment of the Sensitizing Potential of a Compound: Breaking Down the *In Vivo* Events

Susan Gibbs and Krista Ouwehand
Department of Dermatology, VU University Medical Centre, Amsterdam, The Netherlands

1. Introduction

Contact dermatitis is a common health problem, which affects both men and women and accounts for 85-90% of all skin diseases. Two main types of contact dermatitis can be distinguished, according to the patho-physiological mechanisms involved, i.e. allergic and irritant contact dermatitis. Allergic contact dermatitis requires the activation of antigen specific (i.e. acquired) immunity leading to the development of effector T cells, which mediate skin inflammation (Nosbaum et al., 2009; Saint-Mezard et al., 2004). Irritant contact dermatitis is due to inflammatory and toxic effects caused by exposure to xenobiotics activating an innate local inflammatory reaction (Mathias and Maibach, 1978; Nosbaum et al., 2009). Identification of a potential sensitizer and its distinction from an irritant substance (non-sensitizer) currently completely relies on animal testing. The mouse Local Lymph Node Assay (LLNA) is the most frequently used and accurate test with regards to relevance (predictive capacity) and reliability (reproducibility within and between laboratories) in distinguishing a sensitizer from a non-sensitizer (Basketter et al., 2007; Gerberick et al., 2005; Kimber, 2002). This is closely followed by the Guinea pig maximization test (Basketter and Scholes, 1992). In Europe as from 2013 animal testing of cosmetic products will be prohibited (Directive 76/768/EEC), while the implementation of the REACH (Registration, Evaluation and Authorization of Chemicals) legislation (European Regulation 2006) will result in an increased demand for risk assessment of nearly 30,000 chemicals already marketed in the EU. Moreover, the replacement, reduction, and refinement of the use of test animals in general is now strongly advocated. Therefore, there is an urgent need for reliable *in vitro* assays, which are able to distinguish sensitizers from non-sensitizers. This chapter describes the progress being made to develop a battery of assays, which mimics human sensitization *in vitro* and therefore which may in the future be able to replace the use of test animals.

In order to develop such a battery of assays it is important to first understand the different *in vivo* events which occur during sensitization. The skin functions as a barrier protecting an individual from dehydration, mechanical trauma, irradiation, microbial insults, and from direct exposure to harmful sensitizing or irritant chemicals (Elias, 2005; Elias, 2007). The barrier function is provided by the uppermost layer of the epidermis, the stratum corneum. The stratum corneum consists of dead, terminally differentiated keratinocytes (corneocytes) embedded in extracellular lipid. The corneocytes and the lipid component of the stratum corneum can be considered as bricks and mortar and form the barrier to the environment and potentially harmful substances (Bouwstra and Ponec, 2006; Elias, 1983; Elias, 2004). In order for a potential sensitizer to cause an allergic reaction it must first penetrate or damage the stratum corneum in order to exert its effect on the viable epidermal and dermal layers below. Once a chemical has penetrated the stratum corneum, it is metabolized by binding to homologous skin proteins. As a result the new antigenic moieties may exert cytotoxic effects on the keratinocytes, and trigger keratinocytes to release alarm signals in the form of cytokines and chemokines. In addition, these hapten-protein complexes may become antigenic for cells of the immune system, such as DC. DC are professional antigen presenting cells, which can efficiently stimulate T cell responses and are therefore important for the initiation and regulation of antigen- or hapten-specific immune responses (Banchereau et al., 2000; Guermonprez et al., 2002; Mellman and Steinman, 2001). In human skin, both epidermal DC (i.e. the Langerhans cells (LC)) as well as dermal DC (DDC) are involved in the initiation of allergic contact dermatitis (Aiba, 2007; Bennett et al., 2005; Kaplan et al., 2005). Following encounter with an allergen, LCs become activated and undergo maturation and differentiate from antigen-capture and processing cells into potent immunostimulatory DCs, able to present antigen effectively to effector T-cells. In order to activate antigen specific acquired immunity leading to the development of effector T-cells, LC migrate to the paracortical area of the regional lymph nodes, where they display the allergenic epitope to naïve T-cells (Aiba et al., 1993; Lanzavecchia and Sallusto, 2001; Nosbaum et al., 2009; Reid et al., 2000; Saint-Mezard et al., 2004). This results in expansion and differentiation of allergen reactive T cells, thereby forming specific effector and memory T cells, which migrate via the efferent lymphatics into the bloodstream and recirculate through the body (Sallusto et al., 1999).

There are a number of considerations which should be taken into account when developing an *in vitro* assay for assessment of the sensitizing potential of a compound. In all cases, for an *in vitro* model to replace an animal model it should be able to distinguish a sensitizer from a non-sensitizer to the same degree as the current animal models. Currently it is thought that no single assay will meet these requirements and therefore a battery of assays should be developed which will be used in a tiered manner. This chapter describes the progress on the development of human *in vitro* assays for assessment of the sensitizing potential of a compound, based on the five crucial *in vivo* events in skin sensitization (Fig. 1):

1. The ability of the chemical to penetrate through the stratum corneum: bioavailability
2. The potential of the chemical to metabolize into stable conjugates to create an immunogenic complex
3. The ability of a chemical to trigger alarm signals from keratinocytes
4. The ability of a chemical to induce maturation and migration of DCs
5. The ability of a chemical to provoke T-cells responses.

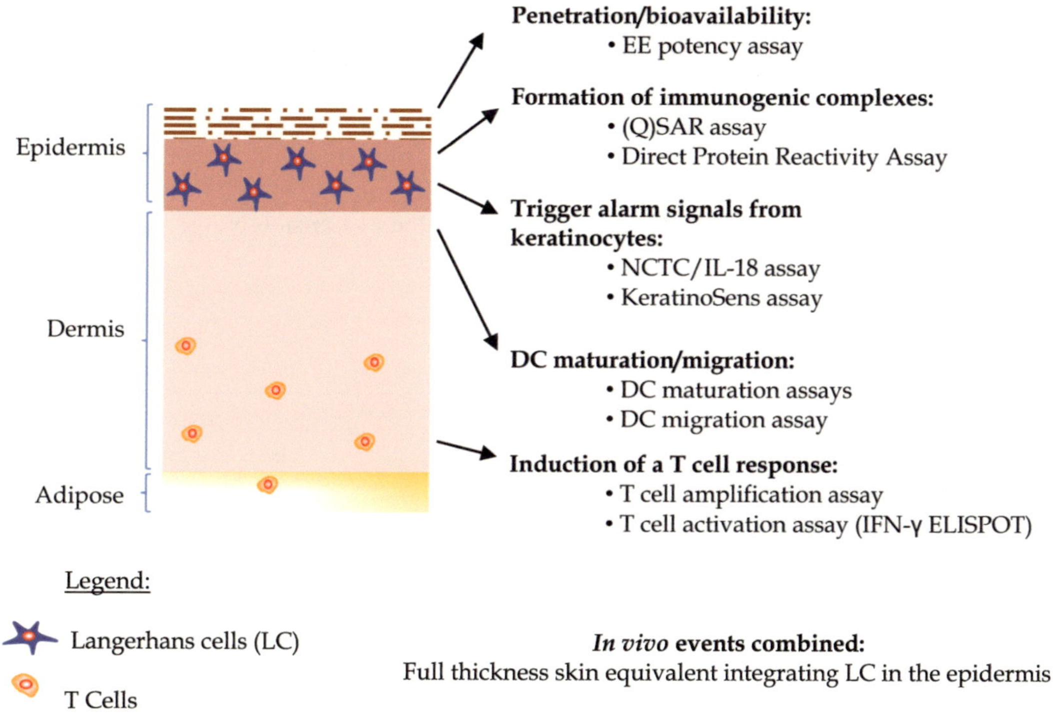

Fig. 1. Assays under development which mimic sensitization *in vitro*

2. *In vitro* assays

2.1 *In vitro* barrier competency

Contact dermatitis is the result of harmful compounds being able to penetrate the skin, to induce either a local inflammation reaction or a delayed hypersensitivity response. One of the most promising alternatives to animal testing for determining whether or not a chemical can penetrate the stratum corneum is an assay which makes use of human reconstructed epidermal equivalent cultures (EE). Indeed an assay using EE has undergone full validation by European Centre for Validation of Alternative Methods (ECVAM) and is now accepted as an animal alternative for identifying potentially irritant or cytotoxic substances (Spielmann et al., 2007).

EE potency assay: Reconstructed EE have a three-dimensional structure which is generated by growing keratinocyte cultures at the air-liquid interface on transwell filters or collagen matrices (Gibbs, 2009). Culture at the air-liquid interface stimulates epidermal differentiation to such a degree that a basal layer, spinous layer, granular layer and most importantly a stratum corneum is formed. A potential assay to determine the potency of a sensitizing chemical is based on that chemical's ability to penetrate the stratum corneum and then to exert an irritant/ cytotoxic effect on the underlying viable keratinocytes within the epidermis. The assay is based on the clinical observation that most sensitizers also have irritant properties and therefore the potency of the sensitizer may be directly related to the potency of the irritant. In this way the EE-EC_{50} value (effective chemical concentration required to reduce cell viability by 50%) is calculated after chemical exposure of EE (Fig. 2). The stronger the sensitizer, the greater its irritant property and therefore the lower the EE-EC_{50} value (Dos Santos et al., 2011; Spiekstra et al., 2009). Since this assay does not distinguish sensitizers from non-sensitizers, its potential application is in a tiered strategy, where tier 1 identifies sensitizers (see below) which are then tested in tier 2, this assay, which determines sensitizer potency. Currently the EE potency assay is undergoing pre-validation in a European ring study in order to determine its transferability, reproducibility and efficacy domain.

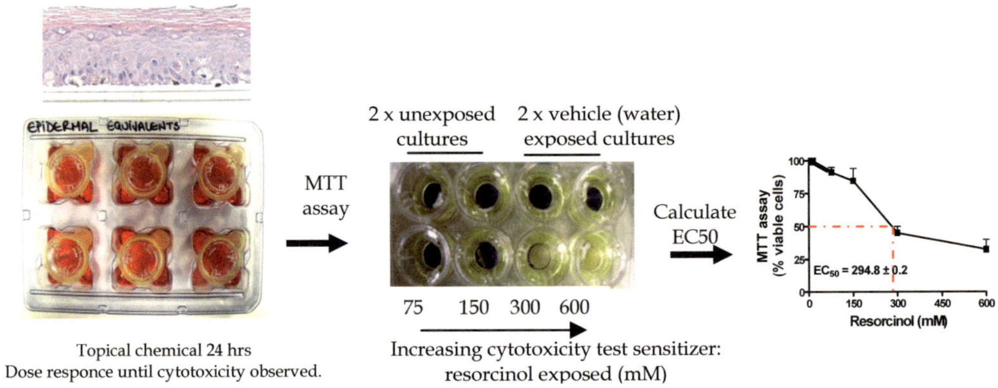

Fig. 2. Epidermal Equivalent potency assay. Left side: EE are cultured air exposed. Each culture has a diameter of 1 cm. Serial dilutions of chemicals are applied topically to the stratum corneum of the EE for 24 hours. Hereafter the MTT assay is performed. Right side: The MTT assay is representative of mitochondrial activity and cell viability and the readout of the assay quantifies dehydrogenase activity. After 24 hour chemical exposure, epidermal equivalents are transferred to new culture plates containing Thiazolyl Blue Tetrazolium Bromide solution which is the substrate for dehydrogenase present within the living cells. After two hours incubated at standard culture conditions, the formed crystals (blue/black in colour) are dissolved in isopropanol / HCl (3:1) solution overnight. Absorbance of the solution is measured at 570 nm and expressed in percentage relative to the absorbance value of vehicle (water) exposed cultures) (Dos Santos et al., 2011; Spiekstra et al., 2009).

2.2 Formation of immunogenic complexes

Following penetration of the skin, haptens reach the viable epidermis where many of the pivotal events and metabolic processes take place. In immunological terms, chemical allergens (haptens) as such are unable to elicit immune responses. For an immune response to be achieved, they must first bind with a protein to form an immunogenic complex. Stable associations between the chemical allergen and proteins/glycoproteins are formed (Karlberg et al., 2008). Such complexes can then interact with epidermal LCs, and probably other cutaneous DCs. Therefore, chemical reactivity is a key parameter in many assays as it is an essential part of sensitization..

(Q)SAR assay: One potential approach to skin sensitization hazard identification is the use of (Quantitative) structure activity relationships ((Q)SARs) coupled with appropriate

documentation and performance characteristics. These (Q)SAR models are extensively reviewed by Patelwicz et al. (Patlewicz et al., 2007). In brief, (Q)SAR models describe the ability of chemicals (haptens) to react with proteins to form covalently-linked conjugates in correlation to their skin sensitization capability. For all such models, there is a need to estimate the hapten–protein interactions. This is done either qualitatively, by evaluating the presence or absence of a specific substructure in a molecule, or quantitatively, by using electronic descriptors for estimating the potential reactivity of a molecule (Patlewicz et al., 2007; Roberts et al., 1983). Other approaches for addressing chemical reactivity aim at determining chemical reactivity towards biologically relevant nucleophiles. Most of these assays monitor either the disappearance of a nucleophile or the formation of an adduct between the electrophile and the nucleophile (reviewed by Gerberick et al. (Gerberick et al., 2008). The mechanism of formation of such adducts could be proposed by their structure and can be deducted from the analytical data.

Direct Protein Reactivity Assay: Another very promising *in vitro* approach is based on the ability of a chemical to react with proteins containing cysteine and lysine thus forming stable (covalent) bonds (Direct Protein Reactivity Assay). This non-cell based assay classifies minimum reactivity as non-sensitizers and low, moderate and high reactivity as sensitizers. Following two rounds of ring trials inter-laboratory reproducibility was acceptable and concordance was 89 % with LLNA (Gerberick et al., 2008).

2.3 Alarm signals generated by keratinocytes

Keratinocytes play a role in all phases of allergic contact dermatitis. They initiate the early secretion of inflammatory cytokines which trigger LC to mature and migrate from the epidermis to the dermis; they play an important role in T-cell trafficking through the height of the inflammatory phase by directly interacting with epidermotrophic T-cells; and they contribute to the resolution phase of allergic contact dermatitis by producing anti-inflammatory cytokines and participating in tolerogenic antigen presentation to effector T-cells (Gober and Gaspari, 2008). Keratinocytes lack antigen presenting capacity. With regards to this book chapter, we will concentrate on their role in sensitization.

NCTC/ IL-18 assay: If an irititant or sensitizer penetrates the skin, it will result in a large number of different cytokines and chemokines being released from kerationocytes. (Spiekstra et al., 2009; Spiekstra et al., 2005). Antonopoulos et al. demonstrated that IL-18 is a key proximal mediator of LC migration and contact hypersensitivity, acting upstream of IL-1β and TNF-α (Antonopoulos et al., 2008). It has been proposed that IL-18 production in human keratinocytes may be a sensitive method to identify contact allergens, discriminating them from respiratory allergens and irritants (Corsini et al., 2009; Galbiati et al., 2011). Results in the human keratinocyte cell line NCTC2455 and primary human keratinocytes, both cultured as a monolayer, show that at non-cytotoxic concentrations (cell viability higher of 75%, as assessed by MTT reduction assay), all contact sensitizers, including pro-haptens, induced a dose-related increase in intra-cellular IL-18, whereas both irritants and respiratory sensitizers did not. This indicates that cell-associated IL-18 may provide an *in vitro* tool for identification and discrimination of contact allergens from respiratory allergens and/or irritants. This NCTC / IL-18 assay is currently undergoing pre-validation in a European ring study in order to determine its transferability, reproducibility and efficacy domain.

The KeratinoSens assay: This assay measures gene-induction events at sub-cytotoxic concentrations, based on the fact that the majority of skin sensitizers induce the Nrf2-Keap1-ARE regulatory pathway (Ade et al., 2009; Andreas et al., 2011; Natsch and Emter, 2008; Vandebriel et al., 2010). The KeratinoSens reporter cell line was made by transfection of human HaCaT keratinocytes with the antioxidant response element (ARE) from the human AKR1C2 gene, which was inserted in front of a SV40 promoter and placed upstream of a luciferase gene. Induction of luciferase in this cell line was used to screen for skin sensitizers, resulting in both qualitative (sensitizer/ non-sensitizer categorization) and quantitative (concentration for significant gene induction) reproduciblity between laboratories (Emter et al., 2010). This extensive KeratoSens ring study involving 5 laboratories tested 28 substances and had an accuracy ranging between 85.7 and 92.9 % in the different laboratories (Andreas et al., 2011).

2.4 DC maturation and migration

Human skin accommodates immature cutaneous dendritic cells, called LC and DDC. Upon allergen exposure of the skin, DCs recognize and internalize the hapten-protein complex, thereby losing their potential to capture new antigens and gain the potential to present the hapten-protein complex to naïve T cells. These changes are commonly known as DC maturation. Simultaneously, under the influence of epidermal cytokines (e.g.: IL-1α, IL-1β, TNF-α, IL-18) and fibroblast-, blood endothelial-, and lymph endothelial-chemokines (CXCL12, CCL19, CCL21), maturing LC migrate from the epidermis to the dermis and then to the draining lymph nodes where they can present the antigen to T-cells (Antonopoulos et al., 2008; Cumberbatch et al., 2003a; Cumberbatch et al., 2001; Cumberbatch et al., 2003b; Enk and Katz, 1992; MartIn-Fontecha et al., 2003; Ouwehand et al., 2008; Villablanca and Mora, 2008). DC activation upon allergen exposure also leads to functional changes in DC, such as alterations in cytokine (TNF-α IL-1β) and chemokine secretion (De Smedt et al., 2002; Toebak et al., 2006a; Toebak et al., 2006b), and to upregulation of chemokine receptors expression (CCR7, CXCR4) (Jugde et al., 2005; Rustemeyer et al., 2003; Staquet et al., 2004). Many co-stimulatory molecules and intercellular adhesion molecules (e.g.: HLA-DR, HLA-ABC, CD40, CD80, CD83, CD86, ICAM-1/CD54) are also upregulated during DC maturation (Aiba et al., 1997; Ozawa et al., 1996; Rambukkana et al., 1995). Together these changes in biomarker expression and migratory properties have been tested in *in vitro* DC based assays in order to distinguish a sensitizer from a non-sensitizer.

DC maturation assays: The maturation of DC upon exposure to contact allergens has been extensively reviewed by Dos Santos et al. (Dos Santos *et al.*, 2009). Both DC derived from fresh blood cell progenitors and DC-like cell lines have been tested. Currently, the secretion of IL-8 (also known as CXCL8) by allergen activated maturing DC appears to be the most promising read-out in order to distinguish a sensitizer from a non-sensitizer in both DC derived from fresh blood cell progenitors and DC-like cell lines (Fig. 3). With the exception of several false positive and negative results, also CD54, CD86 and p38 mitogen activated protein kinase (MAPK) upregulation could distinguish most sensitizers from non-sensitizers. Based on these studies, the h-CLAT (Ashikaga et al., 2010; Ashikaga et al., 2006) and MUSST *in vitro* assays (Klein and Reek, 2000), which measure surface marker expression in THP-1 and U-937 cells, respectively, have entered pre-validation. When comparing with the U-937 and THP-1 ring studies each involving 2 laboratories testing 6 sensitizers, 3 non-sensitizers and combined assessment of CD86 and CD54, the THP-1 assay showed a 100 % inter-laboratory accuracy and the U-937 assay showed a 67 % inter-laboratory accuracy (Sakaguchi et al., 2006).

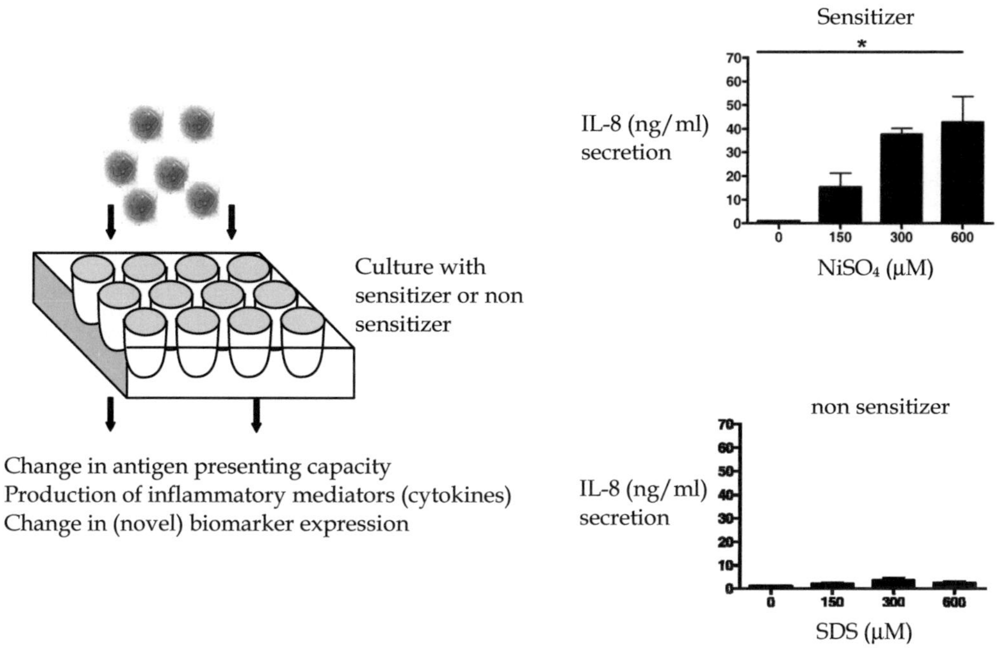

Fig. 3. Dendritic cell biomarker assay. DC (cell line MUTZ-3) are exposed for 24 hours to sensitizer $NiSO_4$ or non-sensitizer SDS. The relative amount of IL-8 secreted after $NiSO_4$ exposure as compared to its solvent control increases with increasing chemical concentrations, while no increase in IL-8 secretion is observed after SDS exposure (Ouwehand et al. 2010b).

DC migation assay: Migration of LC is associated with an increase in CXCR4 and a decrease in CCR1/ CCR3/ CCR5 receptors (Lin et al., 1998; Neves et al., 2008) on the maturing LC's combined with an increase in the secretion of the chemokine CXCL12 (ligand for CXCR4) in the dermis from fibroblasts (Fig. 4). The increase in CXCL12 secretion by fibroblasts is a general stress signal since it is induced by TNF-α (Ouwehand et al., 2008) and in burns (Avniel et al., 2006) and is therefore not restricted to sensitizers. The mature LC's eventually travel in a CXCR4 / CCR7 dependent manner to the lymph nodes where they may prime T cells resulting in sensitization (Villablanca and Mora, 2008). In contrast to sensitizer mediated LC migration via the CXCR4 / CXCL12 axis, non-sensitizer (irritant) mediated LC migration is mediated by maintained CCR1/ CCR3/ CCR5 (not decreased) expression and low CXCR4 expression on immature LC together with upregulated CCL5 secretion by dermal fibroblasts. Increased levels of CCL5 result in drawing CCR1/ CCR3/ CCR5 expressing LC from the epidermis into the dermis (Ouwehand et al., 2010a). The DC migration assay is based on the differential chemokine receptor expression on LC after exposure to sensitizers (CXCR4) or non-sensitizers (CCR1, CCR3 and/or CCR5) and their ability therefore to migrate preferentially to CXCL12 or CCL5 respectively (Fig. 4). This

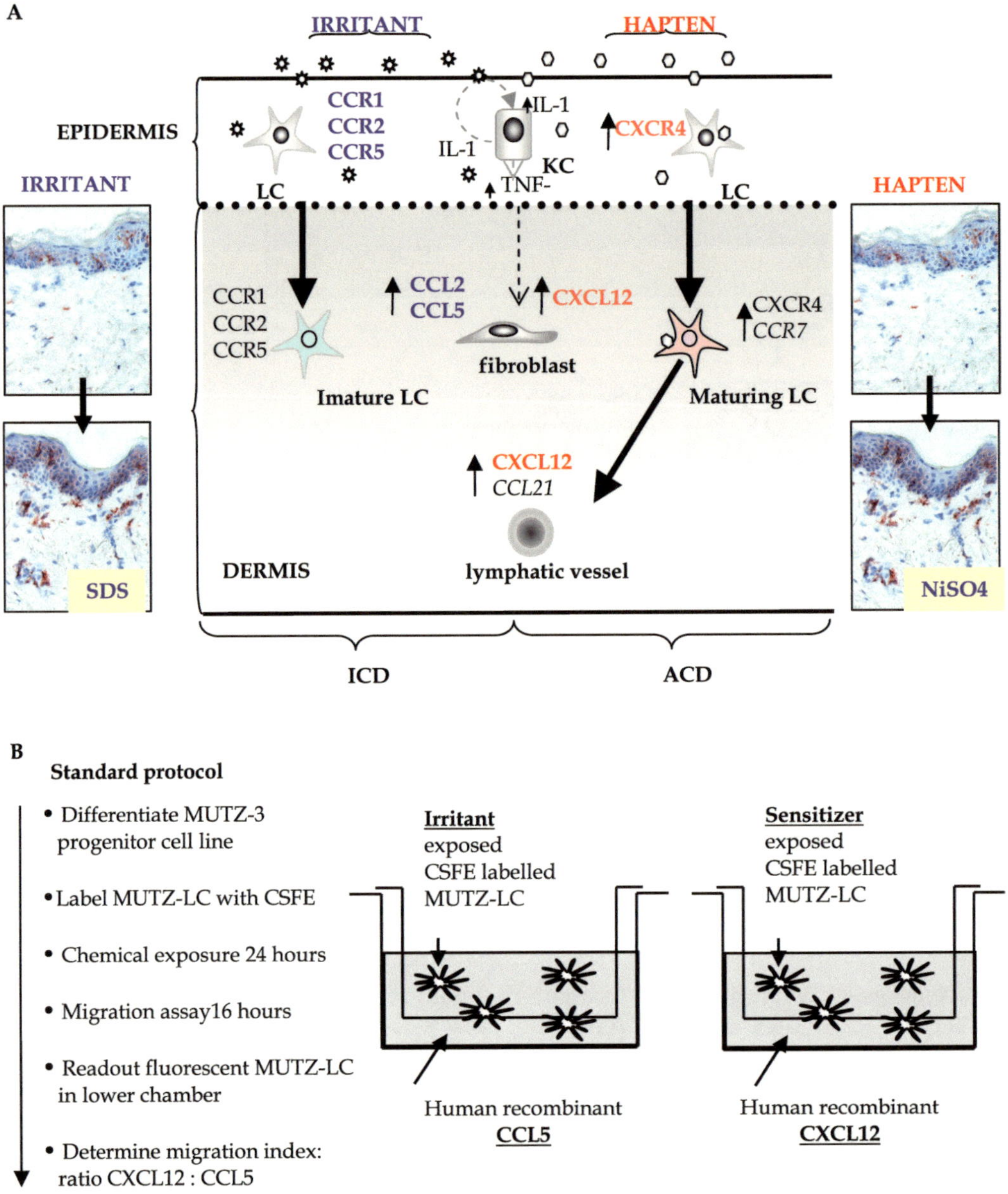

Fig. 4. A: Mechanism of Langerhans cell migration after sensitizer (hapten) or irritant exposure. Full thickness skin was exposed to $NiSO_4$ (sensitizer), or SDS (irritant) for 16 h. Cryosections were prepared and immuno-stained for the characteristic LC marker CD1a (Magnification 200x). Upon exposure to both sensitizer and irritant a decrease in LC (red stained cells) number could be observed in the epidermis and a subsequent increase in LC number was found in the dermis, as compared to the vehicle control (Ouwehand et al., 2008; 2010a).
B: Protocol for DC migration assay. The number of MUTZ-LC migrating towards either rhCXCL12 or rhCCL5 in the transwell assay system is expressed as a CXCL12/CCL5 ratio. A CXCL12/CCL5 ratio above 1 is indicative of a sensitizer, whereas a CXCL12/CCL5 ratio below 1 is indicative of a non-sensitizer (Ouwehand et al., 2010b).

assay uses MUTZ-3 cell line derived LCs (MUTZ-LC). MUTZ-LC exposed to non-cytotoxic concentrations of sensitizers (including pro-haptens) in the upper chamber of a transwell migrate towards CXCL12 in the lower transwell chamber, whereas MUTZ-LC exposed to non-sensitizers in the upper chamber of a transwell migrate towards CCL5 in the lower transwell chamber (Ouwehand et al., 2010b). The read-out of the assay is the relative number of fluorescent MUTZ-LC entering the lower chamber expressed as a ratio of CXCL12 : CCL5. A ratio > 1 indicates that the chemical is a sensitizer whereas a ratio < 1 indicates that the chemical is a non-sensitizer. This assay has been tested in a ring-study, whereby three different European laboratories have shown that the assay is transferable. Intra-laboratory and inter-laboratory variation with regards to MUTZ-3 progenitor culture, differentiation to MUTZ-LC, maturation and assay implementation showed that results were consistent between the laboratories, and the dose response data was reproducible in the three laboratories (Rees et al. tox. In Vitro. In press).

2.5 Induction of a T cell response

T cell assays: The induction of T cell responses to chemicals, drugs and protein allergens is the key event that decides whether sensitization will lead to manifestation of disease. Therefore, T cell assays despite their complexity can support and improve risk assessment and hazard identification strategies. Test chemicals can be added either directly to the T cells or as hapten-protein conjugates. Alternatively, chemicals can also be used to modify DC, which in turn present the hapten protein-complex to T cells. The current status on T cell assays has recently been reviewed (Martin et al., 2010). Typically, two readout systems are used:

1. T cell proliferation using radioactive labeling or dilution fluorochromes such as carboxyfluorescein succinimidyl ester (CFSE).
2. T cell activation markers, such as CD137, CD154 (CD40L), and IFN-γ to identify antigen-activated T cells (Frentsch et al., 2005; Wehler et al., 2008).

In order to increase the sensitivity of the system, these methods may be combined with a polyclonal T cell amplification step before the addition of specific allergen (Geiger et al., 2009). These assays could help in predictive risk assessment and hazard identification as they may address the induction of innate immune responses. Because of the need to work with primary cells in an autologous setting, due to differences in individual TCR repertoires, these assays are not expected to be used for high throughput screening, but may be suitable a tiered approach, in order to predict the immunological effect of a chemical.

2.6 Skin equivalents integrating DC

Full thickness skin equivalent integrating LC in the epidermis: The five crucial steps involved in sensitization could in principle be investigated using freshly excised human skin, as this is physiologically the most relevant model to study the human skin immune defence system. However, a major drawback of using excised skin for screening purposes is the regular need for large amounts of fresh skin, which potentially creates logistical obstacles and high donor variation. Alternatively, an *in vitro* fully integrated model containing defined cell types (e.g. keratinocytes, melanocytes, fibroblasts, LC, and T cells) from allogeneic sources or cell lines, would reduce the donor variability and logistical obstacles experienced by using freshly excised human skin for in vitro assays. Several attempts have been made in order to develop such an *in vitro* skin equivalent (SE) model. Currently, only two groups have succeeded in introducing LC into an EE (Facy et al., 2004; Facy et al., 2005; Regnier et al., 1997; Schaerli et al., 2005), while just one group was able to introduce dendritic cells (DC) into a dermal equivalent (Guironnet et al., 2001). Neither of these groups reconstructed a full-thickness SE, rendering these models unfit to study all processes involved in the development of a hypersensitivity reaction. Three groups have so far succeeded in reconstructing a full thickness SE containing keratinocytes, fibroblasts, and epidermal LC containing Birbeck granules (Bechetoille et al., 2007; Dezutter-Dambuyant et al., 2006; Ouwehand et al., 2011). The model described by Ouwehand et al. is the only one to use cell line derived LC (MUTZ-3 derived LC) which overcomes the logistical problems of using fresh donor derived LC progenitors from peripheral blood or cord blood (Ouwehand et al., 2011). Importantly this model was shown to be functional and suited to study the first four steps in the development of an allergic response since topical exposure to sensitizers resulted in MUTZ-LC maturation and migration into the dermis (Ouwehand et al., 2011). However, no models until date contain T cells, rendering them unsuitable to study the induction of T cell responses to chemicals. In the future these models may progress to co-culture with T cells in the lower compartment of the transwell system. A shortcoming of the models that require fresh blood-derived precursor cells as their source of LC would be the logistics involved in constructing an autologous T cell containing co-culture variant (Dezutter-Dambuyant et al., 2006). The model of Ouwehand contains a human LC cell line (MUTZ-3 derived LC), established from the peripheral blood of a HLA-A2 positive patient with acute myelomonocytic leukemia (Ouwehand et al., 2011). These MUTZ-LC were able to prime specific and fully functional CTL from HLA-A2-matched healthy donors (Santegoets et al., 2008), which reduce logistical problems created by the need for blood of healthy volunteers. For all of these integrated skin models, further research is required to determine whether they will contribute to the battery of assays being developed for risk assessment. In any case, these models are excellent to study DC biology *in vitro*.

3. Conclusions

As the induction of contact hypersensitivity is the result of a series of parallel and sequential processes, it is thought that a battery of assays based on the *in vivo* events leading up to sensitization will be required to identify potential sensitizers *in vitro*. Such a battery of assays would be expected to reduce the risk of scoring false negatives and positives. There is a general consensus that a combination of several functionally distinct human-based *in vitro* assays will be successful and may eventually even surpass the accuracy of animal methods such as LLNA. Several mechanistically relevant and promising test-strategies are being developed, which need to be further refined and tested before entering formal validation according to the guidelines of the European Centre for the Validation of Alternative Methods to animal testing (ECVAM). Although recent developments are looking very promising, scientists will find it difficult to meet the 2013 European deadline for replacement of animal based methods with *in vitro* alternatives.

4. References

Ade, N.; Leon, F.; Pallardy, M.; Peiffer, J.L.; Kerdine-Romer, S.; Tissier, M.H.; Bonnet, P.A.; Fabre, I.; Ourlin, J.C. (2009). *HMOX1 and NQO1 genes are upregulated in response to contact sensitizers in dendritic cells and THP-1 cell line: role of the Keap1/Nrf2 pathway.* Toxicol Sci 107:451-460.

Aiba, S.(2007). *Dendritic cells: importance in allergy.* Allergol Int 56:201-208.

Aiba, S.; Nakagawa, S.; Ozawa, H.; Miyake, K.; Yagita, H.; Tagami, H. (1993). *Up-regulation of alpha 4 integrin on activated Langerhans cells: analysis of adhesion molecules on Langerhans cells relating to their migration from skin to draining lymph nodes.* J Invest Dermatol 100:143-147.

Aiba, S.; Terunuma, A.; Manome, H.; Tagami, H. (1997). *Dendritic cells differently respond to haptens and irritants by their production of cytokines and expression of co-stimulatory molecules.* Eur J Immunol 27:3031-3038.

Antonopoulos, C.; Cumberbatch, M.; Mee, J.B.; Dearman, R.J.; Wei ,X.Q.; Liew, F.Y.; Kimber, I. Groves, R.W. (2008). *IL-18 is a key proximal mediator of contact hypersensitivity and allergen-induced Langerhans cell migration in murine epidermis.* J Leukoc Biol 83:361-367.

Ashikaga, T.; Sakaguchi, H.; Sono, S.; Kosaka, N.; Ishikawa, M.; Nukada, Y.; Miyazawa, M.; Ito, Y.; Nishiyama, N.; Itagaki, H. (2010). *A comparative evaluation of in vitro skin sensitisation tests: the human cell-line activation test (h-CLAT) versus the local lymph node assay (LLNA).* Altern Lab Anim 38:275-284.

Ashikaga, T.; Yoshida, Y.; Hirota, M.; Yoneyama, K.; Itagaki, H.; Sakaguchi, H.; Miyazawa, M.; Ito, Y.; Suzuki, H.; Toyoda, H. (2006). *Development of an in vitro skin sensitization test using human cell lines: the human Cell Line Activation Test (h-CLAT). I. Optimization of the h-CLAT protocol.* Toxicol In Vitro 20:767-773.

Avniel, S.; Arik, Z.; Maly, A.; Sagie, A.; Basst, H.B.; Yahana, M.D.; Weiss, I.D.; Pal, B.; Wald, O.; Ad-El, D.; Fujii, N.; Renzana-Seisdedos, F.; Jung, S.; Galun, E.; Gur, E.; Peled, A. (2006). *Involvement of the CXCL12/CXCR4 pathway in the recovery of skin following burns.* J Invest Dermatol 126:468-476.

Banchereau, J.; Briere, F.; Caux, C.; Davoust, J.; Lebecque, S.; Liu, Y.J.; Pulendran, B.; Palucka, K. (2000). *Immunobiology of dendritic cells.* Annu Rev Immunol 18:767-811.

Basketter, D.A.; Gerberick, F.; Kimber, I. (2007). *The local lymph node assay and the assessment of relative potency: status of validation.* Contact Dermatitis 57:70-75.

Basketter, D.A.; Scholes, E.W. (1992). *Comparison of the local lymph node assay with the guinea-pig maximization test for the detection of a range of contact allergens.* Food Chem Toxicol 30:65-69.

Bechetoille, N.; Dezutter-Dambuyant, C.; Damour, O.; Andre, V.; Orly, I.; Perrier, E. (2007). *Effects of solar ultraviolet radiation on engineered human skin equivalent containing both Langerhans cells and dermal dendritic cells.* Tissue Eng 13:2667-2679.

Bennett, C.L.; van, R.E.; Jung, S.; Inaba, K.; Steinman, R.M.; Kapsenberg, M.L.; Clausen, B.E. (2005). *Inducible ablation of mouse Langerhans cells diminishes but fails to abrogate contact hypersensitivity.* J Cell Biol 169:569-576.

Bouwstra, J.A.; Ponec, M. (2006). *The skin barrier in healthy and diseased state.* Biochim Biophys Acta 1758:2080-2095.

Corsini, E.; Mitjans, M.; Galbiati, V.; Lucchi, L.; Galli, C.L.; Marinovich, M. (2009). *Use of IL-18 production in a human keratinocyte cell line to discriminate contact sensitizers from irritants and low molecular weight respiratory allergens.* Toxicol In Vitro 23:789-796.

Cumberbatch, M.; Bhushan, M.; Dearman, R.J.; Kimber, I.; Griffiths, C.E. (2003a). *IL-1beta-induced Langerhans' cell migration and TNF-alpha production in human skin: regulation by lactoferrin*. Clin Exp Immunol 132:352-359.

Cumberbatch, M.; Dearman, R.J.; Antonopoulos, C.; Groves, R.W.; Kimber, I. (2001). *Interleukin (IL)-18 induces Langerhans cell migration by a tumour necrosis factor-alpha- and IL-1beta-dependent mechanism.* Immunology 102:323-330.

Cumberbatch, M.; Dearman, R.J.; Griffiths, C.E.; Kimber, I. (2003b). *Epidermal Langerhans cell migration and sensitisation to chemical allergens.* APMIS 111:797-804.

De Smedt, A.C.; Van Den Heuvel, R.L.; Van Tendeloo, V.F.; Berneman, Z.N.; Schoeters, G.E.; Weber, E.; Tuschl, H. (2002). *Phenotypic alterations and IL-1beta production in CD34(+) progenitor- and monocyte-derived dendritic cells after exposure to allergens: a comparative analysis.* Arch Dermatol Res 294:109-116.

Dezutter-Dambuyant, C.; Black, A.; Bechetoille, N.; Bouez, C.; Marechal, S.; Auxenfans, C.; Cenizo, V.; Pascal, P.; Perrier, E.; Damour, O. (2006). *Evolutive skin reconstructions: from the dermal collagen-glycosaminoglycan-chitosane substrate to an immunocompetent reconstructed skin.* Biomed Mater Eng 16:85s-94s.

Dos Santos, G.G.; Reinders, J.; Ouwehand, K.; Rustemeyer, T.; Scheper, R.J.; Gibbs, S. (2009). *Progress on the development of human in vitro dendritic cell based assays for assessment of the sensitizing potential of a compound.* Toxicol Appl Pharmacol 236:372-382.

Dos Santos, G.G.; Spiekstra, S.W.; Sampat-Sardjoepersad, S.C.; Reinders, J.; Scheper, R.J.; Gibbs, S. (2011). *A potential in vitro epidermal equivalent assay to determine sensitizer potency.* Toxicol In Vitro 25:347-357.

Elias, P.M. (1983). *Epidermal lipids, barrier function, and desquamation.* J Invest Dermatol 80:44s-49s.

Elias, P.M. (2004). *The epidermal permeability barrier: from the early days at Harvard to emerging concepts.* J Invest Dermatol 122:36-39.

Elias, P.M. (2005). *Stratum corneum defensive functions: an integrated view.* J Invest Dermatol 125:183-200.

Elias, P.M. (2007). *The skin barrier as an innate immune element.* Semin Immunopathol 29:3-14.

Emter, R.; Ellis, G.; Natsch, A. (2010). *Performance of a novel keratinocyte-based reporter cell line to screen skin sensitizers in vitro.* Toxicol Appl Pharmacol 245:281-290.

Enk, A.H.; Katz, S.I. (1992). *Early events in the induction phase of contact sensitivity.* J Invest Dermatol 99:39s-41s.

Facy, V.; Flouret, V.; Regnier, M.; Schmidt, R. (2004). *Langerhans cells integrated into human reconstructed epidermis respond to known sensitizers and ultraviolet exposure.* J Invest Dermatol 122:552-553.

Facy, V.; Flouret ,V.; Regnier, M.; Schmidt, R. (2005). *Reactivity of Langerhans cells in human reconstructed epidermis to known allergens and UV radiation.* Toxicol In Vitro 19:787-795.

Frentsch, M.; Arbach, O.; Kirchhoff ,D.; Moewes, B.; Worm, M.; Rothe, M.; Scheffold, A.; Thiel, A. (2005). *Direct access to CD4+ T cells specific for defined antigens according to CD154 expression.* Nat Med 11:1118-1124.

Galbiati, V.; Mitjans, M.; Lucchi, L.; Viviani, B.; Galli, C.L.; Marinovich, M.; Corsini ,E. (2011). *Further development of the NCTC 2544 IL-18 assay to identify in vitro contact allergens.* Toxicol In Vitro 25:724-732.

Geiger, R.; Duhen, T.; Lanzavecchia, A.; Sallusto, F. (2009). *Human naive and memory CD4+ T cell repertoires specific for naturally processed antigens analyzed using libraries of amplified T cells.* J Exp Med 206:1525-1534.

Gerberick, F.; Aleksic, M.; Basketter, D.; Casati, S.; Karlberg, A.T.; Kern, P.; Kimber, I.; Lepoittevin, J.P.; Natsch, A.; Ovigne, J.M.; Rovida, C.; Sakaguchi, H.; Schultz, T. (2008). *Chemical reactivity measurement and the predicitve identification of skin sensitisers. The report and recommendations of ECVAM Workshop 64.* Altern Lab Anim 36:215-242.

Gerberick, G.F.; Ryan, C.A.; Kern, P.S.; Schlatter, H.; Dearman, R.J.; Kimber, I.; Patlewicz, G.Y.; Basketter, D.A. (2005). *Compilation of historical local lymph node data for evaluation of skin sensitization alternative methods.* Dermatitis 16:157-202.

Gibbs, S. (2009). In *vitro irritation models and immune reactions.* Skin Pharmacol Physiol 22:103-113.

Gober, M.D.; Gaspari, A.A. (2008). *Allergic contact dermatitis.* Curr Dir Autoimmun 10:1-26.

Guermonprez, P.; Valladeau, J.; Zitvogel, L.; Thery, C.; Amigorena, S. (2002). *Antigen presentation and T cell stimulation by dendritic cells.* Annu Rev Immunol 20:621-667.

Guironnet, G.; Dezutter-Dambuyant, C.; Gaudillere, A.; Marechal,S.; Schmitt, D.; Peguet-Navarro, J. (2001). *Phenotypic and functional outcome of human monocytes or monocyte-derived dendritic cells in a dermal equivalent.* J Invest Dermatol 116:933-939.

Jugde, F.; Boissier, C.; Rougier-Larzat, N.; Corlu, A.; Chesne, C.; Semana, G.; Heresbach, D. (2005). *Regulation by allergens of chemokine receptor expression on in vitro-generated dendritic cells.* Toxicology 212:227-238.

Kaplan, D.H.; Jenison, M.C.; Saeland, S.; Shlomchik, W.D.; Shlomchik, M.J. (2005). *Epidermal langerhans cell-deficient mice develop enhanced contact hypersensitivity.* Immunity 23:611-620.

Karlberg, A.T.; Bergstrom, M.A.; Borje, A.; Luthman, K.; Nilsson, J.L. (2008). *Allergic contact dermatitis--formation, structural requirements, and reactivity of skin sensitizers.* Chem Res Toxicol 21:53-69.

Kimber, I. (2002). *Reduction, refinement and replacement: putting the immune system to work.* Altern Lab Anim 30:569-577.

Klein, H.U.; Reek, S. (2000). The *MUSTT study: evaluating testing and treatment.* J Interv Card Electrophysiol 4 Suppl 1:45-50.

Lanzavecchia, A.; Sallusto, F. (2001). *The instructive role of dendritic cells on T cell responses: lineages, plasticity and kinetics.* Curr Opin Immunol 13:291-298.

Lin, C.L.; Suri, R.M.; Rahdon, R.A.; Austyn, J.M.; Roake, J.A. (1998). *Dendritic cell chemotaxis and transendothelial migration are induced by distinct chemokines and are regulated on maturation.* Eur J Immunol 28:4114-4122.

Martin, S.F.; Esser, P.R.; Schmucker, S.; Dietz, L.; Naisbitt, D.J.; Park, B.K.; Vocanson, M.; Nicolas, J.F.; Keller, M.; Pichler, W.J.; Peiser, M.; Luch, A.; Wanner, R.; Maggi, E.; Cavani, A.; Rustemeyer, T.; Richter, A.; Thierse, H.J.; Sallusto, F. (2010). *T-cell recognition of chemicals, protein allergens and drugs: towards the development of in vitro assays.* Cell Mol Life Sci 67:4171-4184.

MartIn-Fontecha, A.; Sebastiani, S.; Hopken, U.E.; Uguccioni, M.; Lipp, M.; Lanzavecchia, A.; Sallusto, F. (2003). *Regulation of dendritic cell migration to the draining lymph node: impact on T lymphocyte traffic and priming.* J Exp Med 198:615-621.

Mathias, C.G.;Maibach, H.I. (1978). *Dermatotoxicology monographs I. Cutaneous irritation: factors influencing the response to irritants.* Clin Toxicol 13:333-346.

Mellman, I.; Steinman, R.M. (2001). *Dendritic cells: specialized and regulated antigen processing machines.* Cell 106:255-258.

Natsch, A.; Caroline, B.; Leslie, F.; Frank, G.; Kimberly, N.; Allison, H.; Heather, I.; Robert, L.; Stefan, O.; Hendrik, R.; Andreas, S.; Roger, E. (2011). *The intra- and inter-laboratory reproducibility and predictivity of the KeratinoSens assay to predict skin sensitizers in vitro: results of a ring-study in five laboratories.* Toxicol In Vitro 25:733-744.

Natsch, A.; Emter, R. (2008). *Skin sensitizers induce antioxidant response element dependent genes: application to the in vitro testing of the sensitization potential of chemicals.* Toxicol Sci 102:110-119.

Neves, B.M.; Cruz, M.T.; Francisco, V.; Goncalo, M.; Figueiredo, A.; Duarte, C.B.; Lopes, M.C. (2008). *Differential modulation of CXCR4 and CD40 protein levels by skin sensitizers and irritants in the FSDC cell line.* Toxicol Lett 177:74-82.

Nosbaum, A.; Vocanson, M.; Rozieres, A.; Hennino, A.; Nicolas, J.F. (2009). *Allergic and irritant contact dermatitis.* Eur J Dermatol 19:325-332.

Ouwehand, K.; Santegoets, S.J.; Bruynzeel, D.P.; Scheper, R.J.; de Gruijl, T.D.; Gibbs, S. (2008). *CXCL12 is essential for migration of activated Langerhans cells from epidermis to dermis.* Eur J Immunol 38:3050-3059.

Ouwehand, K.; Scheper, R.J.; de Gruijl, T.D.; Gibbs, S. (2010a). *Epidermis-to-dermis migration of immature Langerhans cells upon topical irritant exposure is dependent on CCL2 and CCL5.* Eur J Immunol 40:2026-2034.

Ouwehand, K.; Spiekstra, S.W.; Reinders, J.; Scheper, R.J.; de Gruijl, T.D.; Gibbs, S. (2010b). *Comparison of a novel CXCL12/CCL5 dependent migration assay with CXCL8 secretion and CD86 expression for distinguishing sensitizers from non-sensitizers using MUTZ-3 Langerhans cells.* Toxicol In Vitro 24:578-585.

Ouwehand, K.; Spiekstra, S.W.; Waaijman, T.; Scheper, R.J.; de Gruijl, T.D.; Gibbs, S. (2011). *Technical Advance: Langerhans cells derived from a human cell line in a full-thickness skin equivalent undergo allergen-induced maturation and migration.* J Leukoc Biol. E-pub ahead of print.

Ozawa, H.; Nakagawa, S.; Tagami, H.; Aiba, S. (1996). *Interleukin-1 beta and granulocyte-macrophage colony-stimulating factor mediate Langerhans cell maturation differently.* J Invest Dermatol 106:441-445.

Patlewicz, G.; Aptula, A.O.; Uriarte, E.; Roberts, D.W.; Kern, P.S.; Gerberick, G.F.; Kimber, I.; Dearman, R.J.; Ryan, C.A.; Basketter, D.A. (2007). *An evaluation of selected global (Q)SARs/expert systems for the prediction of skin sensitisation potential.* SAR QSAR Environ Res 18:515-541.

Rambukkana, A.; Bos, J.D.; Irik, D.; Menko, W.J.; Kapsenberg, M.L.; Das, P.K. (1995). *In situ behavior of human Langerhans cells in skin organ culture.* Lab Invest 73:521-531.

Regnier, M,; Staquet, M.J.; Schmitt, D.; Schmidt, R. (1997). *Integration of Langerhans cells into a pigmented reconstructed human epidermis.* J Invest Dermatol 109:510-512.

Reid, S.D.; Penna, G.; Adorini, L. (2000). *The control of T cell responses by dendritic cell subsets.* Curr Opin Immunol 12:114-121.

Roberts, D.W.; Goodwin, B.F.; Williams, D.L.; Jones, K.; Johnson, A.W.; Alderson, J.C. (1983). *Correlations between skin sensitization potential and chemical reactivity for p-nitrobenzyl compounds.* Food Chem Toxicol 21:811-813.

Rustemeyer, T.; Preuss, M.; von Blomberg, B.M.; Das, P.K.; Scheper, R.J. (2003). *Comparison of two in vitro dendritic cell maturation models for screening contact sensitizers using a panel of methacrylates.* Exp Dermatol 12:682-691.

Saint-Mezard, P.; Rosieres, A.; Krasteva, M.; Berard, F.; Dubois, B.; Kaiserlian, D.; Nicolas, J.F. (2004). *Allergic contact dermatitis.* Eur J Dermatol 14:284-295.

Sakaguchi, H.; Ashikaga, T.; Miyazawa, M.; Yoshida, Y.; Ito, Y.; Yoneyama, K.; Hirota, M.; Itagaki, H.; Toyoda, H.; Suzuki, H. (2006). *Development of an in vitro skin sensitization test using human cell lines; human Cell Line Activation Test (h-CLAT). II. An inter-laboratory study of the h-CLAT.* Toxicol In Vitro 20:774-784.

Sallusto, F.; Kremmer, E.; Palermo, B.; Hoy, A.; Ponath, P.; Qin, S.; Forster, R.; Lipp, M.; Lanzavecchia, A. (1999). *Switch in chemokine receptor expression upon TCR stimulation reveals novel homing potential for recently activated T cells.* Eur J Immunol 29:2037-2045.

Santegoets, S.J.; Bontkes, H.J.; Stam, A.G.; Bhoelan, F.; Ruizendaal, J.J.; van den Eertwegh, A.J.; Hooijberg, E.; Scheper, R.J.; de Gruijl, T.D. (2008). *Inducing antitumor T cell immunity: comparative functional analysis of interstitial versus Langerhans dendritic cells in a human cell line model.* J Immunol 180:4540-4549.

Schaerli, P.; Willimann, K.; Ebert, L.M.; Walz, A.; Moser, B. (2005). *Cutaneous CXCL14 targets blood precursors to epidermal niches for Langerhans cell differentiation.* Immunity 23:331-342.

Spiekstra, S.W.; Dos Santos, G.G.; Scheper, R.J.; Gibbs, S. (2009). *Potential method to determine irritant potency in vitro - Comparison of two reconstructed epidermal culture models with different barrier competency.* Toxicol In Vitro 23:349-355.

Spiekstra, S.W.; Toebak, M.J.; Sampat-Sardjoepersad, S.; van Beek, P.J.; Boorsma, D.M.; Stoof, T.J.; von Blomberg, B.M.; Scheper, R.J.; Bruynzeel, D.P.; Rustemeyer, T.; Gibbs, S. (2005). *Induction of cytokine (interleukin-1alpha and tumor necrosis factor-alpha) and chemokine (CCL20, CCL27, and CXCL8) alarm signals after allergen and irritant exposure.* Exp Dermatol 14:109-116.

Spielmann, H.; Hoffmann, S.; Liebsch, M.; Botham, P.; Fentem, J.H.; Eskes, C.; Roguet, R.; Cotovio, J.; Cole, T.; Worth, A.; Heylings, J.; Jones, P.; Robles, C.; Kandarova, H.; Gamer, A.; Remmele, M.; Curren, R.; Raabe, H.; Cockshott, A.; Gerner, I.; Zuang, V. (2007). *The ECVAM international validation study on in vitro tests for acute skin irritation: report on the validity of the EPISKIN and EpiDerm assays and on the Skin Integrity Function Test.* Altern Lab Anim 35:559-601.

Staquet, M.J.; Sportouch, M.; Jacquet, C.; Schmitt, D.; Guesnet, J.; Peguet-Navarro, J. (2004). *Moderate skin sensitizers can induce phenotypic changes on in vitro generated dendritic cells.* Toxicol In Vitro 18:493-500.

Toebak, M.J.; Moed, H.; von Blomberg, M.B.; Bruynzeel, D.P.; Gibbs, S.; Scheper, R.J.; Rustemeyer, T. (2006a). *Intrinsic characteristics of contact and respiratory allergens influence production of polarizing cytokines by dendritic cells.* Contact Dermatitis 55:238-245.

Toebak, M.J.; Pohlmann, P.R.; Sampat-Sardjoepersad, S.C.; von Blomberg, B.M.; Bruynzeel, D.P.; Scheper, R.J.; Rustemeyer, T.; Gibbs, S. (2006b). *CXCL8 secretion by dendritic cells predicts contact allergens from irritants.* Toxicol In Vitro 20:117-124.

Vandebriel, R.J.; Pennings, J.L.; Baken, K.A.; Pronk, T.E.; Boorsma, A.; Gottschalk, R.; Van Loveren, H. (2010). *Keratinocyte gene expression profiles discriminate sensitizing and irritating compounds.* Toxicol Sci 117:81-89.

Villablanca, E.J.; Mora, J.R. (2008). *A two-step model for Langerhans cell migration to skin-draining LN.* Eur J Immunol 38:2975-2980.

Wehler, T.C.; Karg, M.; Distler, E.; Konur, A.; Nonn, M.; Meyer, R.G.; Huber, C.; Hartwig, U.F.; Herr, W. (2008). Rapid identification and sorting of viable virus-reactive CD4(+) and CD8(+) T cells based on antigen-triggered CD137 expression. J Immunol Methods 339:23-37.

Part 4

Allergic Contact Dermatitis to Specific Allergens

6

Dental Metal Allergy

Maki Hosoki and Keisuke Nishigawa
The University of Tokushima Graduate School
Japan

1. Introduction

Dental metal allergy is the general term used to describe allergic diseases caused by reactions to dental metal materials. Recently, allergic symptoms involving other dental materials, such as organic compounds, have been reported, and these allergic diseases need to be referred to as either a dental allergy or dental material allergy. When safety evaluations involving biomaterials are performed, various kinds of risk factors, including the potential for cytotoxicity and/or allergization, need to be taken into consideration (Geurtsen, 2002, Wataha, 2000).

At the present time, even ordinal dental treatment requires the use of many kinds of metallic and organic materials, some of which are known to cause allergic symptoms. The first clinical cases of dental metal allergy involved a mercurial allergy to intraoral amalgam fillings that led to stomatitis and dermatitis around the anus (Fleischmann, 1928). Previous studies in many countries have reported a variety of symptoms to be associated with different metals (Hubler&Hubler, 1983, Lundstrom, 1984, Magnusson et al., 1982, Wiesenfeld et al., 1984). Nickel, chromium, mercury, palladium, and cobalt are typical of metals used in dentistry that have caused allergies, which have included reactions to these materials not only in the mucosa of the oral cavity, but also on the skin of the hands, feet, and/or entire body (Gawkrodger, 2005, Hamano et al., 1998, Yanagi et al., 2005).

Typical allergies reported to be associated with dental materials have included contact dermatitis, systemic contact dermatitis, and contact dermatitis syndrome. Since most of the intraoral dental materials cannot be removed from home environments, these allergic reactions tend to be intractable, with repetitions of symptomatic treatments, such as external medications, found in many of these cases. Sometimes general and local dermatitis is found in the skin apart from the intraoral dental material, and it exhibits pathognomonic symptoms of the allergy that are different from those noted in other contact dermatitis.

2. Epidemiology

The prevalence of dental metal allergy has gradually increased over the last decade (Fig. 1). The demography of the dental metal allergy patients who visited Tokushima University Hospital is seen in Table 1. During July 2000 to June 2005, a total of 148 out of 212 patients (69.8%) exhibited a positive allergic reaction to at least one kind of the patch-test reagents. Since more than 80% of these patients were referred from dentists and dermatologists at other medical institutions, we expected to find a higher positive reaction rate as compared to that of the other studies. Over a five-year surveillance period, nickel, palladium, chromium, cobalt and stannum exhibited the highest positive reaction rates to the patch tests in these patients. During this time period, the increases in the positive reaction rates for nickel, palladium, chromium and molybdenum were greater than those seen in our previous study (Fig. 2). (Hosoki et al., 2009)

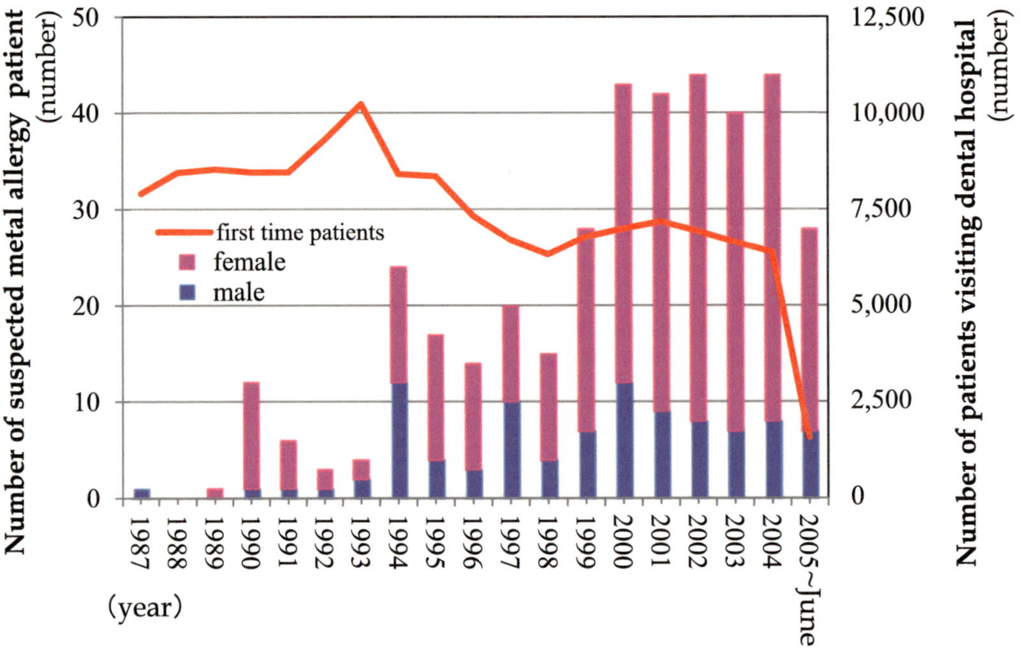

Fig. 1. Number of patients with dental metal allergy.

Period	July 2000 to June 2005	July 1995 to June 2000	July 1987 to June 1995
Patient number	212	114	60
Positive (adjusted residual)	148 (+2.4)	60 (-3.2)	41 (+0.7)
Negative (adjusted residual)	64 (-2.4)	54 (+3.2)	19 (-0.7)
Positive rate (%)	69.80	52.60	68.90

Table 1. Positive patch-test rates.

Akyol et al. have reported on the results of a European standard series of patch tests performed on 1038 contacts dermatitis patients. A total of 32.3% appeared to have a positive reaction with more than one reagent, and nickel exhibited the highest positive reaction rate (17.6%) (Akyol et al., 2005). Lam et al. investigated 2585 contact dermatitis patients and found that 54.7% exhibited a positive reaction rate, with the highest result seen for nickel (24.4%). In 2008, Lam et al. confirmed these results (Lam et al., 2008). On the other hand, Khamaysi et al. reported patch-test results for 121 patients and showed there was a higher positive reaction rate for gold-sodium-thiosulphate (14.0%), nickel sulfate (13.2%), mercury (9.9%), palladium chloride (7.4%), and cobalt chloride (5.0%) (Khamaysi et al., 2006).

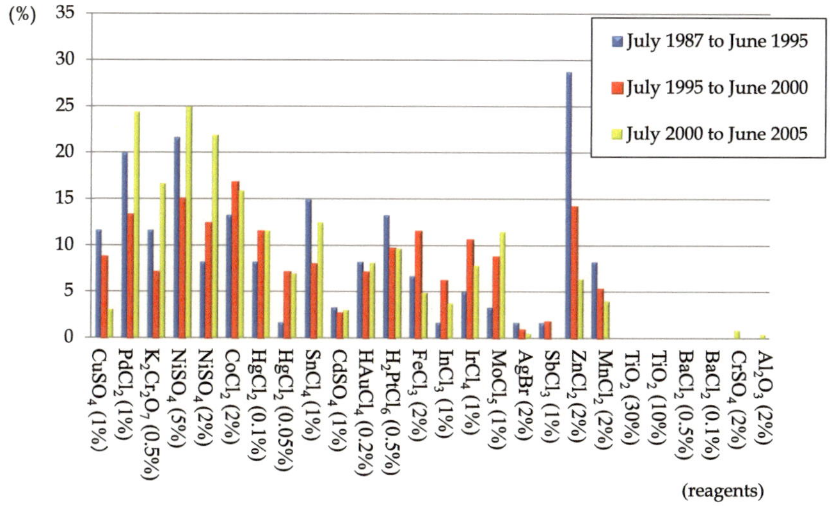

Fig. 2. Positive reaction rates for all patch-test reagents.

There have only been a few studies that examined healthy volunteers and the prevalence of metal allergies. Inoue used 18 types of metal reagents (Patch test allergens metal series, Tori Pharmaceutical Co., Ltd., Japan) to investigate allergic reactions in 1035 adult volunteers. Based on the International Contact Dermatitis Research Group (ICDRG) criteria, Inoue determined that 3.9% of the volunteers (male, 2.7%; female, 4.0%) exhibited positive reactions, regardless of the reagent used. Higher reaction rates were observed for metal reagents that contained $HgCl_2$ (11.1%), $SnCl_2$ (6.3%), $CoCl_2$ (5.4%), and $K_2Cr_2O_7$ (5.1%) (Inoue, 1993). However, since this study was reported in 1993, the estimation of the prevalence rate of metal allergy at present time would be expected to be higher.

3. Pathogenic mechanism

In general, the pathogenic mechanism for metal allergy has been classified as a type IV allergic reaction, which is the same as that for ordinal contact dermatitis (Fisher, 1973). In some cases it has been reported that removal of intraoral dental material containing allergy-positive metal elements relieves atopic dermatitis and asthma symptoms. Thus, this indicates that metal allergies may contain an aspect of the pathogenic mechanism for type I allergic reactions (Hosoki et al., 2002, Nakayama, 2002).

Under normal conditions, chemically stable metallic material rarely causes allergic symptoms. In the human body, the metallic ion itself cannot act as an allergen. However, if an electron from the external shell of a metallic item is removed, then the ionized metal element can be released within the human body. In such cases, these metal elements can bind to protein and form a hapten, which is then recognized by T-cells, and thus, ultimately leads to an allergic reaction (Davies et al., 1977, Ishii et al., 1990). Therefore, the tendency for ionization can be very influential with regard to the creation of an allergic reaction. If this potential ionization of a metal element can be prevented, the risk of metal allergy can be decreased. Unfortunately, intraoral circumstances, such as large amounts of electrolytic solutions, i.e. saliva, always surround metallic restorations and thus, the pH of a solution can rapidly fluctuate in line with the type of diet followed. Overall, this increases the difficulty in preventing changes of the dental metal material that can initiate allergies.

4. Pathology

4.1 Symptoms

Table 2 lists the symptoms and diagnosis of the metal allergy patients who visited the Clinic of Dental Metal Allergy at Tokushima University Hospital during the period ranging from 1987 to 2005. Symptom locations can vary from being on only a limited area of the body, such as on the oral mucosa, hands, palm, back or neck, to being found over the entire skin surface. However, each of these metal elements does not possess a distinct pathology and no correlation has been noted between the class of metal elements and the clinical symptoms. Explanations for the typical symptoms noted for dental metal allergy are presented in the following table.

	Number of patients					
	July 2000 to June 2005		July 1995 to June 2000		July 1987 to June 1995	
Symptoms	Number	%	Number	%	Number	%
Pustulosis palmaris et plantaris/dyshidrotic eczema	51	24.1	19	21.7	9	15.0
Lichen planus	24	11.3	15	17.1	4	6.7
Stomatitis/cheilitis/gingivitis	21	9.9	13	14.8	8	13.3
Contact dermatitis	18	8.5	37	42.2	17	28.3
Allergic rhinitis	10	4.7			1	1.7
Anthema in hands and plantae	10	4.7	2	2.3		
Glossalgia	8	3.8			8	13.3
Asthma	8	3.8			1	1.7
Urticaria	8	3.8	1	1.1		
Atopic dermatitis	7	3.3	12	13.7		
Candidiasis	7	3.3				
Redness and eczema in one hand	7	3.3	2	2.3	3	5.0
Anthema	7	3.3				
Generalized eczema	7	3.3				
Contact dermatitis and redness with pierced earring, ring and necklaces	6	2.8				
Redness (hands and feet/face)	5	2.4				
Intraoral white lesion	4	1.9				
Glossitis/lingual nervous feeling	4	1.9	2	2.3	4	6.7
Solar dermatitis	4	1.9			2	3.3
Other	40	18.9	11	12.5	3	5.0

Table 2. Typical symptoms and diagnoses.

4.2 Pustulosis palmaris et plantaris, and dyshidrotic eczema

In these patients, erythema, blisters with pustules, scale and crust typically appear on the palm and plantar (Fig. 3). In addition, sterile pustules are sometimes accompanied by itch, heat and painful sensations, and on occasion, osteoarthritis may also be found. Osteoarthritis symptoms involve the trunk, peripheral nerves, and the extra-articular region, and frequently there is local swelling, tenderness, heat sensation, and flare noted in these patients. During the early stages, histological findings show there is lymphocyte infiltration into the epidermis along with spongy degeneration. After formation of blisters and at the point where the blister reaches the horny cell layer, neutrophils appear and pustule development begins. At the present time, detailed pathoetiology of these symptoms has yet to be reported. Focal infection of the chronic inflammation from the palatine tonsil, marginal and periapical periodontitis, and metal allergy are all suspected as being predisposing factors.

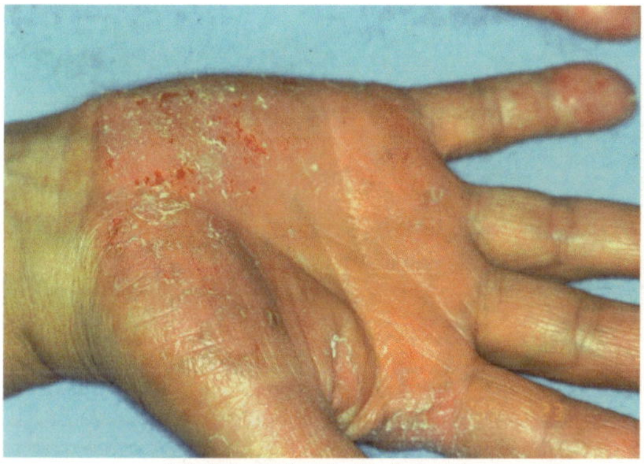

(a) Pustulosis Palmaris

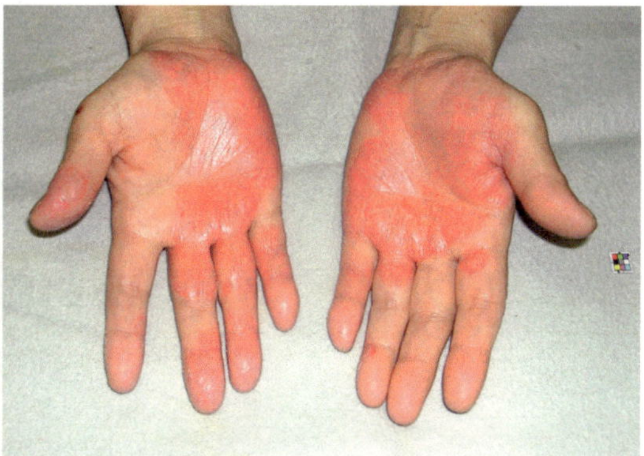

(b) Pustulosis Palmaris

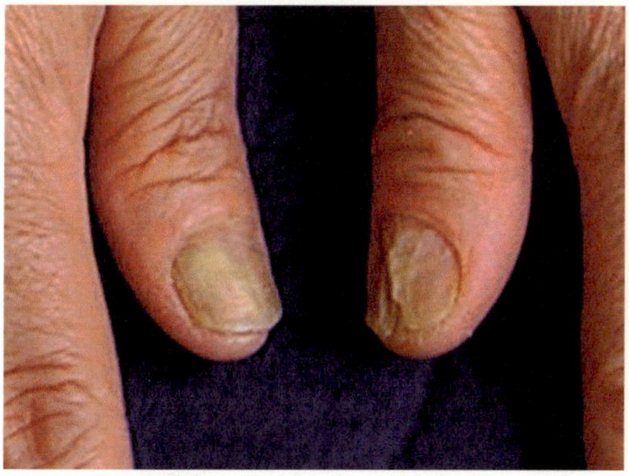

(c) Pustulosis Palmaris (crooked nails)

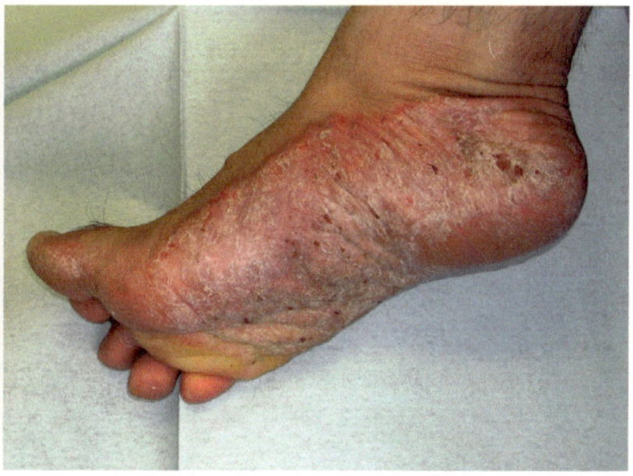

(d) Pustulosis Plantaris

Fig. 3. Pustulosis palmaris et plantaris and dyshidrotic eczema.

4.3 Lichen planus

Chronic inflammatory disease can include dyskeratosis of the skin, oral and external genitalia mucosa. When it appears on the oral mucosa, lace or stitch pattern keratinizations may be present and accompanied by erosion and ulceration (Fig. 4). On the skin, red or purple-red papules are seen at the internal area of the joint extremities and trunk. While some of these papules may be painless, others can cause itch, heat sensation or pain.

The buccal mucosa is the favorite site of lichen planus. In longstanding cases, this keratinization pattern can sometimes spread into the entire oral mucosa. In dental metal allergy cases, it appears at the oral mucosa attached to the metal restoration that contains the allergy-positive metal element.

Histological findings exhibit parakeratosis, liquefaction degeneration of the basal cell, and T lymphocyte infiltration under the epithelial tissue. At the present time, the pathoetiology of lichen planus is still not clear. Mechanical stimulation, metal allergy, and the hepatitis C virus (HCV) are all suspected as being predisposing factors. Since Jubert et al. reported that about 30% of these patients exhibit HCV antibody, inveterate cases of lichen planus should have both liver function and HCV antibody tests performed.

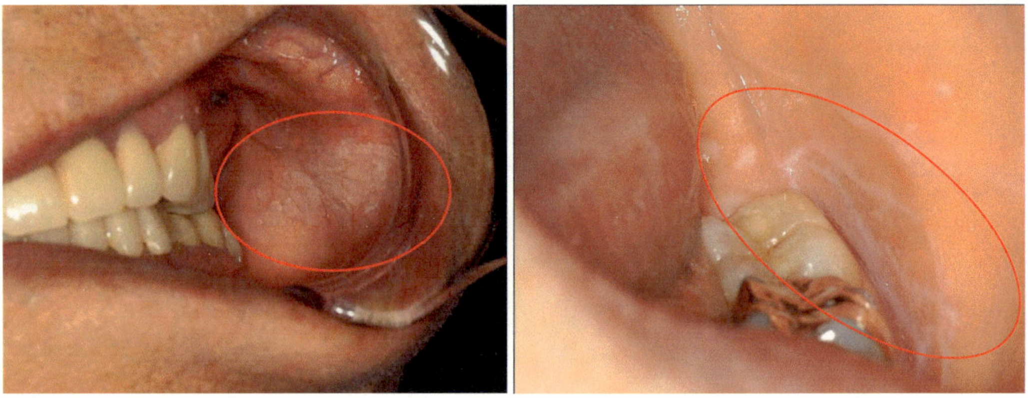

Fig. 4. Lichen planus.

4.4 Stomatitis, glossitis, cheilitis

The clinical and histological findings of these symptoms around the oral cavity do not differ from ordinal oral inflammations. Red halo glossitis and cheilitis sometimes can occur on the

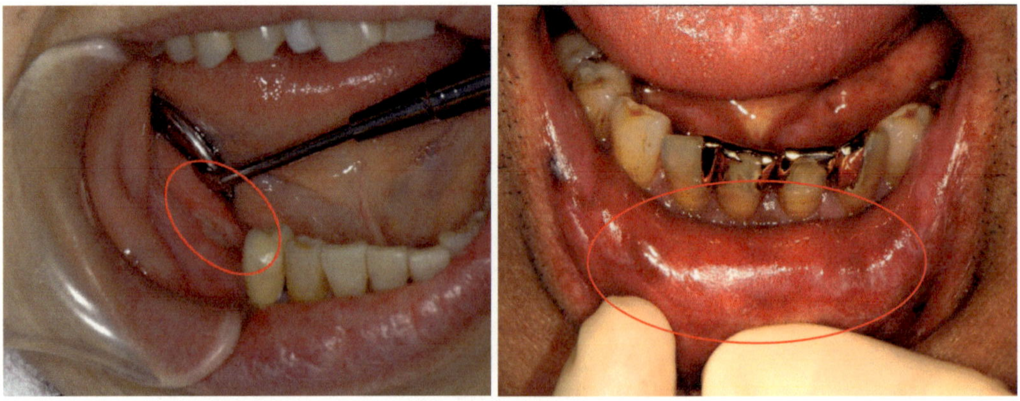

Fig. 5. Stomatitis and cheilitis.

oral mucosa close to the suspected dental prosthesis that contains the allergy-positive metal elements (Fig. 5). However, stomatitis and aphthous oral ulcers can sometimes occur on oral regions that are distant from the dental metal prosthesis. Regardless of the location, recurrent formations of the inflammation are frequently observed in these cases.

4.5 Glossodynia

In glossodynia, the main symptoms that patients encounter are pain, twitching and a burning sensation in the tongue. In some cases, no clear organic changes are ever found. Flare of the tongue, and an atrophy of the filiform papillae similar to that seen in geographical tongue can be found (Fig. 6). Possible predisposing factors include psychological factors, galvanic current, mechanical stimulation, allergy to metal elements eluted from a dental prosthesis, or a shortage of an essential nutrient.

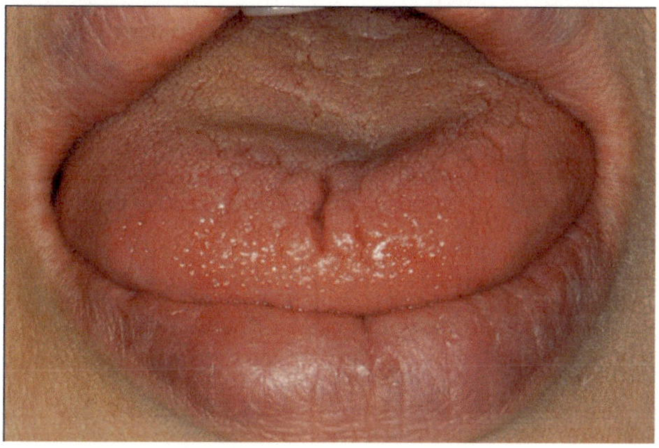

Fig. 6. Glossodynia.

4.6 Generalized eczema and pseudoatopic dermatitis

In generalized eczema, an intractable itching dermatitis occurs on all of the skin (Fig. 7). In 1965, Shanon (Shanon, 1965) first reported pseudoatopic dermatitis to be a general eczematoid dermatitis caused by a chromic allergy due to shoe leather and cement. The clinical findings for this type of dermatitis are exactly the same as those seen for atopic

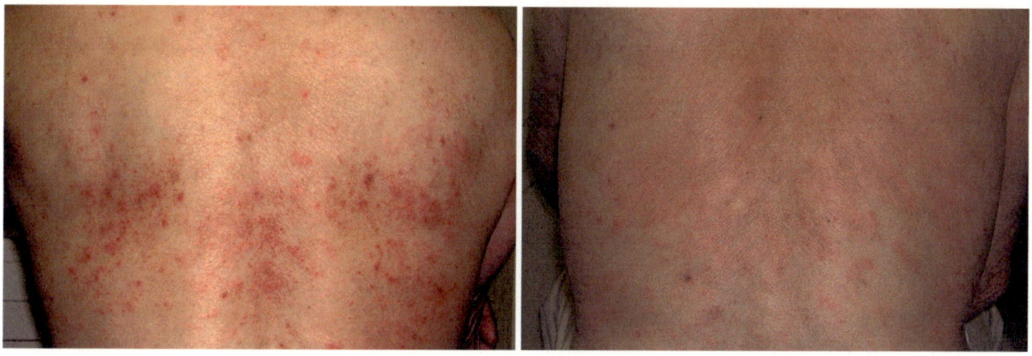

Fig. 7. Generalized eczema and pseudoatopic dermatitis.

dermatitis, with patients exhibiting no atopic diathesis and a low value for the immunoglobulin E (IgE) radioimmunosorbent test. Absorbed allergen is spread by blood flow and causes the eczema and urticaria on general skin, and in some cases is associated with itching, heat and painful sensations. Instead of referring to this as generalized eczema, the symptoms for this could be referred to as atopic dermatitis with metal allergy. The name of this disease is still being debated at the present time.

4.7 Atopic dermatitis

Typical symptoms of atopic dermatitis are chronic eczema with an itching sensation. Serum IgE is generally increased in these patients, and there is a repeated advancement to remission of the symptoms. Intractable cases sometimes exhibit a positive reaction to a metal reagent when using the patch test. In such cases, removing the intraoral metal restorations that contain the allergy-positive metal could lead to a remission of the symptoms. Since the skin barrier function of atopic dermatitis patients is compromised and not enough to prevent infection and sensitization, metal allergies tend to complicate these types of cases.

5. Diagnosis and treatment

The figure shows the flow chart for the diagnosis and treatment of dental metal allergy.

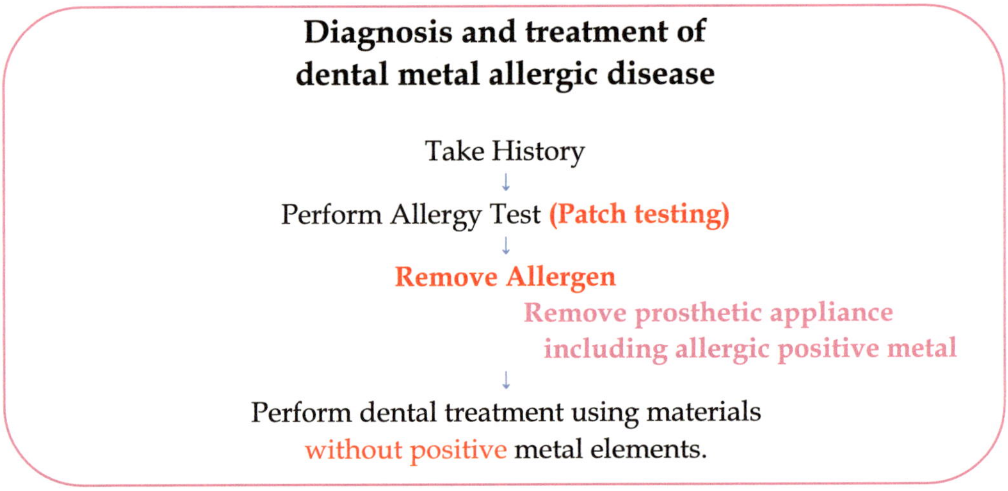

Fig. 8. Flow chart for diagnosis and treatment of dental metal allergic disease.

5.1 History taking

The primary goal of the questions for the metal allergy patients is to obtain a past history concerning their reaction to the metallic items that might be responsible for the allergic reaction. The following case highlights the information that leads to suspecting the patient of having a dental metal allergy.

1. Having incurable skin trouble with red spots, eczema, and vesicles, with ineffective dermatological treatment.
2. React to metals in ornaments and daily necessities, and is hard to cure.

3. After dental treatment with metal material, skin and intraoral symptoms developed or became incurable.

All of the patients were given recommendations to undergo a patch test for the purpose of diagnosing dental metal allergy. As an alternative in vitro examination, lymphocyte activation tests can also be used. However, since lymphocyte activation tests are not available for every metal element, the patch test should be considered as the first choice for confirmation of the diagnosis.

5.2 Patch test

Patch testing should be done according to criteria from the International Contact Dermatitis Research Group (ICDRG). Examination plasters containing the test reagent were attached to the back or the arm of the patient for 48 hours (Groot, 2008). After waiting for one hour after the plaster removal and the effect of the stimulation was gone, changes on the skin surface were evaluated according to the ICDRG criteria (Jean-Marie Lachapelle&Maibach, 2009). The same evaluations were repeated 72 hours and one week later. Since some of the metal reagents tended to exhibit a high reaction 7 days after plaster attachment, a minimum of a one-week test period is required for these tests (Davis et al., 2008). In addition, since aluminum in the Finn Chamber reacts with Hg^{2+} and produces hydrochloric acid, this chamber cannot be used for the $HgCl_2$ reagent.

5.2.1 Metal reagents

The following metal reagents are the primary reagents used for a patch test (Table. 3).

Product name	Test reagent
Trolab Patch Test Allergens	Metal Compounds
Brial Allergen GmbH	Epicutaneous contact allergens
	Dental materials
Chemotechnique Diagnostics	Patch Test Products, Dental Screening DS-1000
	Dental Materials Patients DMP-1000
Torii Patch Test Allergens	Metal series

Table 3. Test reagents

5.3 Treatment of dental metal allergy

If patients exhibited positive reactions to any of the metal reagents of the patch test, intraoral restorations that could potentially contain metal elements should be examined. Since most of the dental metal material is an alloy metal, simply inspecting the material is not adequate for distinguishing the metal elements. Thus, a non-invasive analysis technique that extracts micro dust from the intraoral restoration and examines it with an Electron Probe Micro-Analyzer (EPMA) or an X-Ray Fluorescence Spectroscopy (XRFS) needs to be performed (Minagi et al., 1999, Suzuki, 1995, Uo&Watari, 2004). For the extraction of metal dust, a tungsten-carbide bur is sometimes used to scrape the metal restoration (Minagi et al., 1999, Suzuki, 1995). However, to ensure there were minimal invasions of the site, we employed the following simple silicone point technique.

1. For each sample, prepare the following material set:

- A disposable polishing point (Super-Snap Mini Point, Shofu Corporation, Kyoto, Japan) (Fig. 9)
- Cellulose tape (Sellotape, Nichiban, Tokyo, Japan)
- Polypropylene film (3520 polypropylene, Spex Chemical Sample Press, Metuchen, NJ, USA)

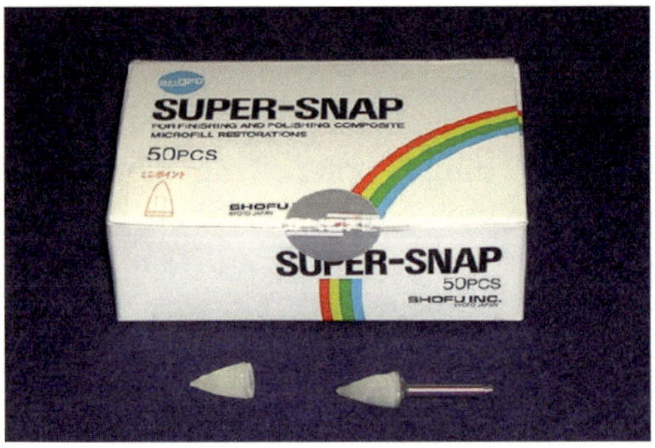

Fig. 9. Disposable polishing point.

2. Clean the surface of the intraoral restoration with a dental cleaning brush in order to remove the plaque and other stains.
3. Attach the Super-Snap to the hand motor and scrub the surface of the metal restoration using a slow speed (1000-2000 rpm). If the antagonistic tooth was restored with a metal material, do not take any samples from the occlusal surface. This will prevent any effect of the metal on the antagonistic tooth.
4. Transfer the metal dust on the surface of the Super-Snap to a cellulose tape strip and cover the tape strip with polypropylene film.
5. The figure below shows pictures of a sample from an intraoral restoration. Micrometal dust on the cellulose tape strip has been covered with polypropylene film. The amount of the extracted sample was about 1 mg and no polishing of the tooth surface was required after the extraction.

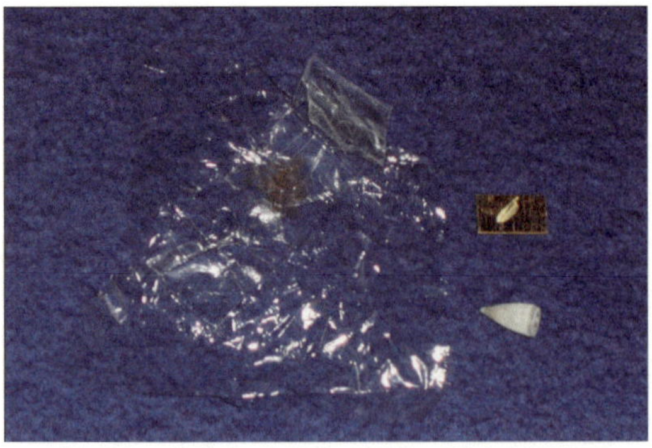

Fig. 10. Polypropylene film, virgin metal sample and a Super-Snap Mini Point.

6. XRF spectroscopy analyzer (EDX900, Shimadzu Corporation, Tokyo, Japan) was used for evaluation of the metal element. Using this analyzer makes it possible for the

acquired sample can be sterilized using gaseous sterilization so that it can then be mailed to facilities that have a micro analyzer (Fig. 11). Since the analysis conditions of the XRFS are different for each device, we have not described the details for each of these devices.

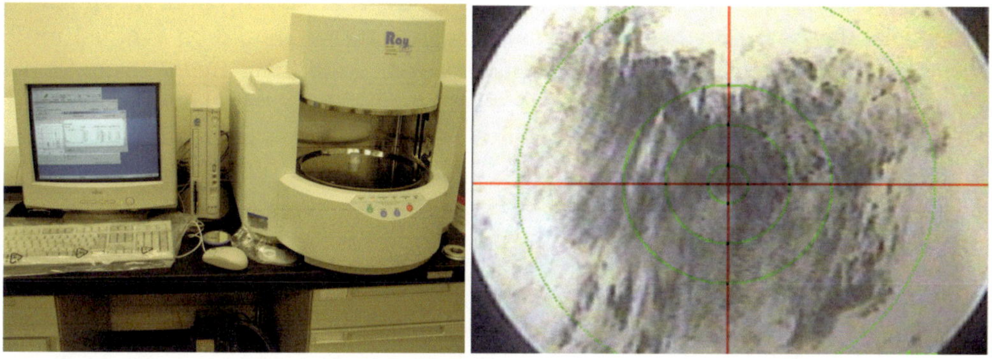

Fig. 11. XRF spectroscopy analyzer and the CCD camera view of the EDX900.

7. Results of the XRF analysis indicated whether or not the intraoral restoration involved an allergy-positive metal element. Since this technique was only available for restorations that were exposed on the surface of a tooth, materials used to build up a tooth, luting cements and root canal fillings could not be examined without having to remove the outer restorations. If the patients are able to identify the dental clinic where the original work was done, then the clinic can be contacted and the name of the metal products used determined before the materials are removed. If information on the actual metal element can be determined, then after informed consent is obtained from the patient, the intraoral metal materials previously utilized can be included in the planning of the subsequent dental treatment to remove the inadequate metal restorations.

5.4 Removal of metal restorations

When removing the restorations that contain allergy-positive metal elements, the removal priority should be as follows.

1. Oral restorations with high elutions, such as black-colored amalgam fillings.
2. Restorations located near the lesion site.
3. Restorations that contain a high rate of allergy-positive metal elements.
4. Two or more restorations with different metal materials that make contact with the occlusion or with the proximal teeth.

In principle, all restorations with allergy-positive metal elements need to be removed. The build-up material that was used for the inside of the full veneer crown is no exception, as it could be eluted. If the patient does not have an allergy to the acrylic material, composite resin filling and/or a temporary restoration with an acrylic resin can be performed to confirm the effect of removing the metallic materials. For patients with an acrylic allergy, glass ionomer cement can be used as a temporary treatment. After the metal material has been removed, sometimes an almost immediate aggravation of the allergic symptoms is observed. This could potentially be due to the effect of metal dust that was swallowed, breathed in, or taken up by the oral mucosa during the removal procedure. In most cases, these symptoms are transient and the patient will recover within a couple of weeks. To avoid the possibility that a patient will develop such symptoms, all metal dust needs to be carefully excluded with oral evacuation equipment along with the adoption of the rubber dam dry field technique, whenever possible. In cases where allergy free metal materials are available, the final prosthesis using such metal material should be avoided until all allergy-positive metal materials have been removed. Additional metal restoration can increase the number of different metal elements in the oral cavity under certain circumstances, which may accelerate the elution of metallic ions from an allergy-positive metal element.

5.5 Reconstruction of dental restorations

Rebuilding of removed restorations should be started after complete elimination of all allergy-positive metal elements and the confirmation of no further relapse of symptoms. New restorations have to be made using allergy-negative materials for each of the individual patients. Since very small amounts of the element could cause an allergic symptom, all materials have to be tested to ensure that every micro component is allergy free. Since the reliability of the patch-test results have not been proven to be perfect, allergy-negative metal elements could still potentially cause allergy symptoms. Thus, during the reconstruction of dental prostheses, the initial restoration should be attached with temporary cement, and the patient prognosis followed for at least one month to ensure there are no allergy symptoms. In the case of a patient with a zinc allergy, careful selection of the luting cement is required. Zinc phosphate, zinc oxide eugenol, polycarboxylate cements along with most of the materials utilized for root canal fillings all have a zinc component and thus, cannot be used.

Lately, there have been many new products for dental restoration that have been developed and introduced in the market. Some of the new products that are listed below might potentially be useful for dental treatments of metal allergy patients.

5.5.1 Titanium

Since titanium possesses a fine biocompatibility property, this material has been used for pacemakers and dental implant biomaterials. Pure titanium can also be used for the material to fabricate a full veneer crown and fixed prostheses of the metal allergy patient. However, it should be noted that titanium wire used for orthodontic treatments contains a nickel-titanium alloy, and is not acceptable for nickel allergy patients.

5.5.2 Highly polymerized compounds

5.5.2.1 Hybrid ceramics

Recent progress of micro fillers and matrix components have greatly improved the physical property of light curing resin products. This newly developed product could potentially be applied in many clinical situations. The following table lists the official properties of the light curing resins currently on the market.

Name (Product)	Filler content (wt%)
Artglass (Heraeus Kulzer)	70
CERAMAGE (SHOFU)	73
GRADIA (GC)	75
ESTENIA C&B (Kuraray)	92
BelleGlass NG (Sybron Dental)	75
Targis (Ivoclar Vivadent)	77
Sculpture (Pentron)	78

Table 4. The official property of hybrid ceramics

5.5.2.2 Rebuilding materials for an abutment tooth

The combination of a composite resin for rebuilding and glass fiber has been used for an alternative to metal core rebuilding. Both a direct and indirect method can be used to fabricate the fibrous post using these materials.

The following are materials that can be used for fibrous posts.

5.5.2.2.1 FiberKor Post system (Pentron Clinical Technologies)

Type S glass fiber (10 μm in diameter) has a high physical property and is bundled up in matrix resin in order to make up the fibrous post used in the rebuilding. Components of the fibrous post are glass fiber (42%), filler (29%) and matrix resin (29%).

5.5.2.2.2 FIBER POST (GC Corp.)

Glass fibers that have a diameter of 14 μm are bundled lengthwise to create high density within the resin matrix. This material contains 58 vol% (77 wt%) of uniformed glass fiber.

5.5.2.2.3 CLEARFIL® FIBER POST (Kuraray)

Premier® Integra Fiber Post (Premier Products Co.)

This product contains 68% pre-silanated Zirconia-rich glass fibers within a composite matrix.

5.5.2.2.4 FRC Postec (Ivoclar Vivadent)

5.5.3 Ceramic materials

The progress in the field of ceramic materials has been quite remarkable as of late. Some of the all-ceramic restoration systems now on the market have a fine biostability and aesthetics that are suitable for use in treating metal allergy patients. With the development of computer-aided design and computer-aided manufacturing (CAD/CAM), all ceramics restorations with aluminous and zirconium coping have become the practical choice for esthetic prostheses (Fig. 12, 13). The zirconium ceramic systems in particular possess fine physical properties with regard to toughness and strength, with some products able to be applied for use in a complete oral reconstruction. The following table lists all of the main ceramic system products that are currently on the market.

Classification by processing		Proprietary name	Product name	Chief ingredient
Slip Technique		In-Ceram Alumina	Vita	Al_2O_3,La_2O_3
		In-Ceram Zilconia	Vita	Al_2O_3, ZrO_2
Press molding		IPS Empress	Ivoclar Vivadent	Leucite
		IPS Empress2	Ivoclar Vivadent	Leucite
		OPC/OPC3G	Pentron	Leucit/Lithium disilicate
		Cergo	Degdent	Leucite
		Finesse All-Ceramic	Dentsply Ceramo	Leucite
Electrophoresis		Wol-Ceramn ELC System	Wol-Dent	Al_2O_3, ZrO_2
CAD/CAM		Cerec	Sirona	Glass ceramics, Llithium disilicate, Polymers
		GN-1	GC	Al_2O_3
		Decsy	Digital process	Leucite
		IPS e.max CAD	Ivoclar Vivadent	Lithium disilicate
CAD/CAM	Yttria	Procera	Nobel Biocare	ZrO_2
		Cercon	DeguDent	ZrO_2
		Lava	3M ESPE	ZrO_2
		Katana	Noritake	ZrO_2
		Everest ZS	KaVo	ZrO_2
		ZENO Zr Discs	WIELAND	ZrO_2
		Aadva Zr	GC	ZrO_2
	Cerium	Nano Zilconia	Panasonic Dental	ZrO_2

Table 5. Ceramic system products

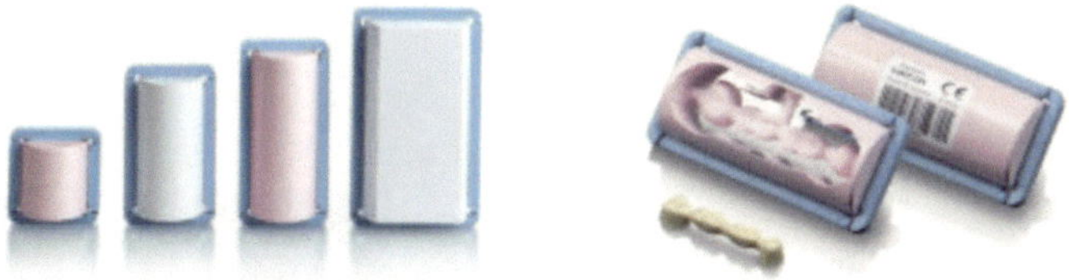

(a) zirconium frame (Cercon, DeguDent)

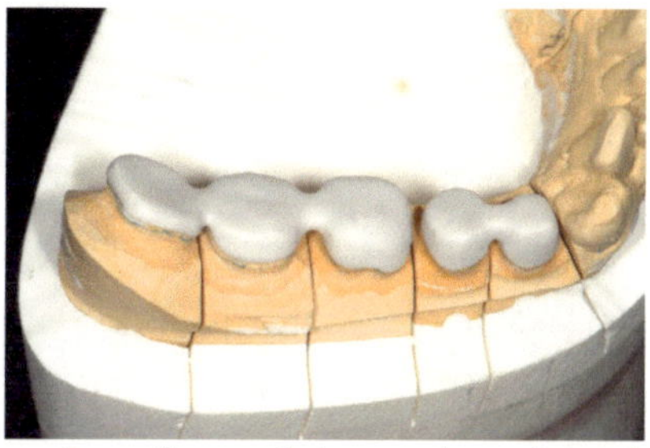

(b) Forming of porcelain on zirconium frame

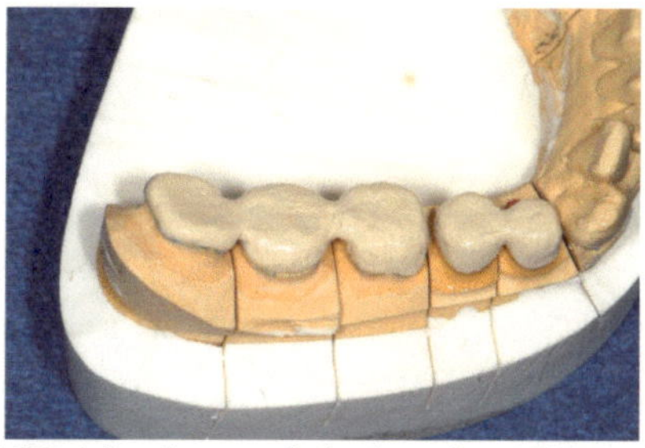

(c) Finished porcelain fused-to-zirconium crowns

Fig. 12. Example of zirconium blocks, zirconium frame before and after the sintering procedure, and the finished all ceramic crown.

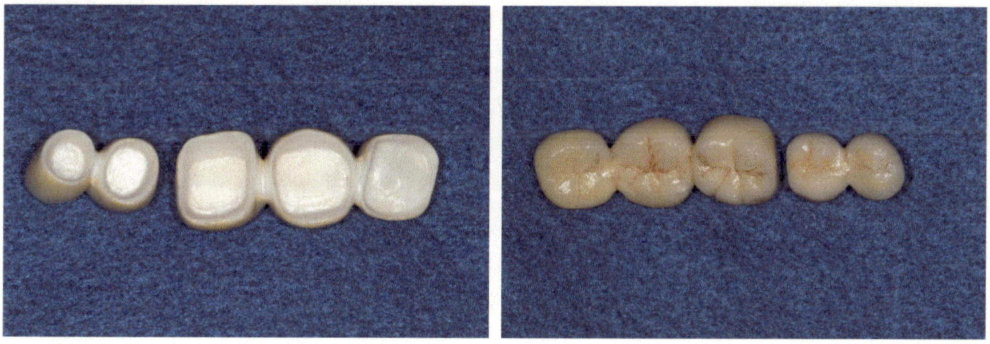

Fig. 13. Example of zirconium crowns.

6. Clinical cases

6.1 Case 1: 51-year-old female with dyshidrotic eczema

The subject was an inpatient of the Dermatological Clinic of Tokushima University Hospital. Results of the patch test at the clinic revealed that the patient had a nickel, cobalt, iridium, zinc, manganese and platinum allergy. The figure 14 shows a picture of the patient's right palm at her initial visit to the Dental Metal Allergy Clinic. Anti-allergic medication and steroid ointment did not result in recovery from her allergic symptoms.

Prognosis

At the time she was seen in the clinic, the zirconium ceramic system for complete oral reconstruction was not on the market. Therefore, a semi-fixed prosthesis with four piece units was designed for maxillary dentition, while a resin clasp denture was fabricated for her missing mandibular molar.

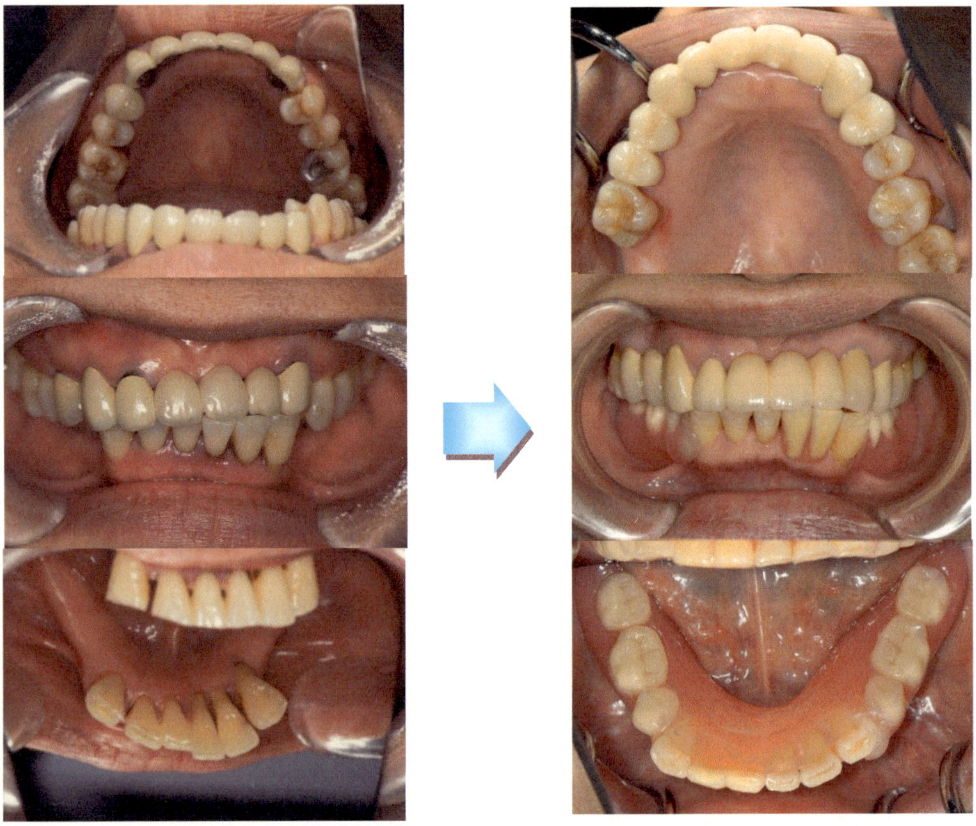

a) Intraoral pictures at first visit (b) Intraoral pictures after dental treatment

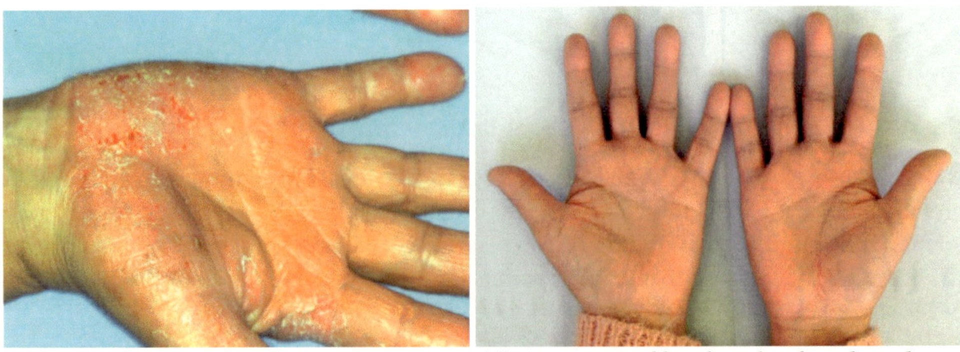

(c) A picture of her hand at first visit (d) A picture of her hands after dental treatment

Fig. 14. Intraoral pictures and hands before and after dental treatment.

6.2 Case 2: 62-year-old male who requested dental implant treatment

This patient had no past history of drug or food allergies and did not have allergic rhinitis. He became aware of his dermatitis symptoms on general skin in 1999 and was given external steroid medications at the dermatology clinic. Since he did not recover from his symptoms, he visited a general hospital in 2000 and was diagnosed with photodermatosis. At the hospital he was administered steroids, but exhibited no remarkable recovery. In 2002, he visited another dermatological clinic and was given external steroids and anti-allergic drugs, however, his symptoms remained. In 2005, he visited Tokushima University Hospital to ask for dental implant treatment. After examination by a dentist, the patient was referred to the Dental Metal Allergy Clinic.

Prognosis

Results of the patch test revealed that the patient had allergy-positive reactions to various kinds of metal reagents. An ultraviolet light test exhibited erythema with more than 5 minutes exposure to ultraviolet A (2.1 J/cm^2) and 50 seconds to ultraviolet B (35 J/cm^2). The

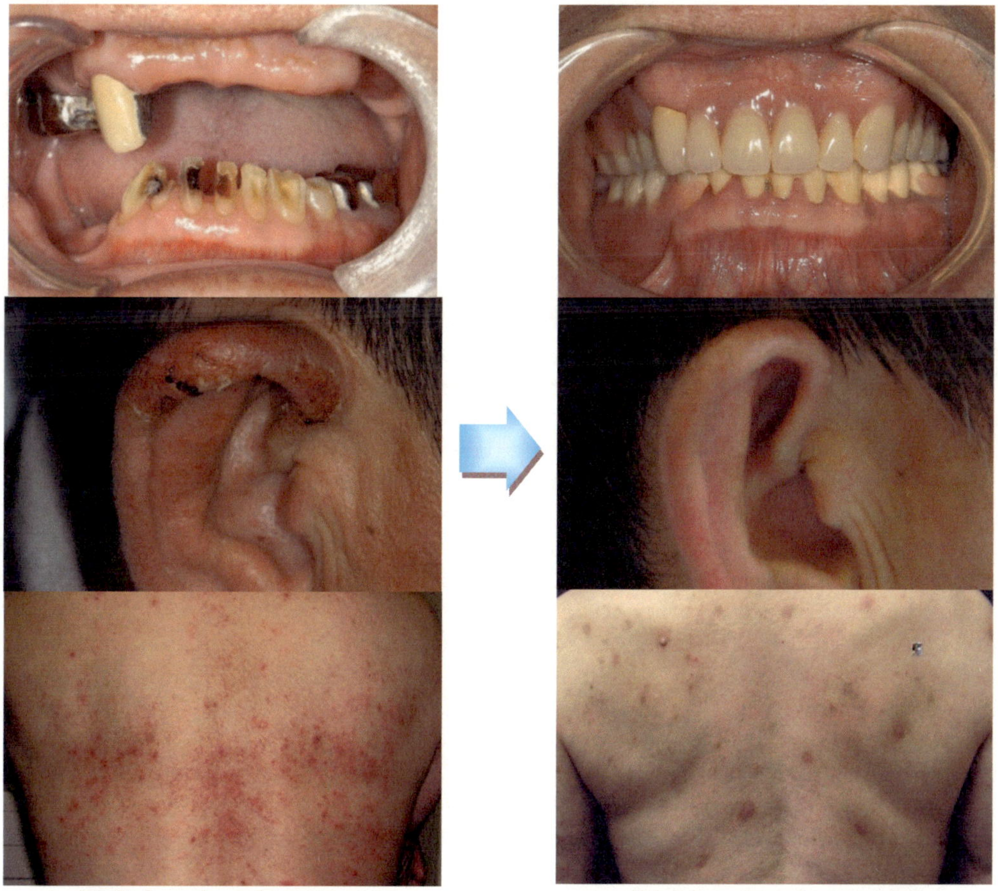

(a) Before dental treatment (b) After dental treatment

Fig. 15. Intraoral picture, and photos of the ear and back before and after the dental treatment.

minimal erythema dose was smaller with ultraviolet A. This patient was diagnosed as having complication dermatitis with photodermatosis, and dental metal allergy.

Subsequently, we then began to remove all metal restorations that contained allergy-positive metal elements. After removal of a fixed prosthesis and extraction of some of his teeth, a removable prosthesis with a non-metal clasp (Jeneric/Pentron, Wallingford, CT, USA) was fabricated. Porcelain fused to zirconium crowns were attached to the patient after complete removal of all of his metal restorations. In conjunction with the progress of the dental treatment, the previously exhibited erythema and swelling gradually reduced, and the prurigo in the local region recovered. The figure 15 shows an intraoral picture and the skin symptoms before and after the dental treatment. Clear recovery of the dermatitis was observed except the neck region that was exposed to sunlight. In this case, the exclusion of the intraoral metal restorations resulted in the healing of the patient's chronic and intractable dermatitis.

7. Discussion

Recently, the number of dental metal allergy patients along with the number of cases that practicing dentists have referred to our special outpatient section have increased. While the cause of this increase is not clear at the present time, suspicions have been raised about the effects of the popularization of pierced earrings as one of the potential causes. In Japan, ear/body piercings since the 1990s have been the cause of nickel allergies in female patients. It is possible that lifestyle choices could be one of the factors responsible for this high prevalence of dental metal allergy. Nickel hypersensitivity is one of the most common metal allergies, and we have documented a high positive reaction rate to nickel reagents. (Hosoki et al., 2009). Larsson-Stymne et al. reported finding a relationship between pierced earrings and nickel allergies (Larsson-Stymne&Widstrom, 1985). Sivertsen et al. also has reported finding the nickel allergy to be associated with pierced ears rather than either local pollution or atopic dermatitis (Smith-Sivertsen et al., 1999). Jensen et al. demonstrated there was a decrease in nickel sensitization in Danish schoolgirls whose ears had been pierced after implementation of the nickel-exposure regulations in 1992 (Jensen et al., 2002). These findings have led to other European countries to regulate exposure to nickel, and in the future, similar regulations may be enacted in Japan. One other study has reported that hypersensitivity reactions to nickel are likely to occur only when there is a prior sensitization from non-dental contacts, and even if this occurs, these sensitizations are still rare (Setcos et al., 2006, Spiechowicz et al., 1999). It is likely that nickel allergens from sources other than dental material will need to be considered in the future, as the use of the nickel alloy in dental materials in Japan is on the wane. Patients with inflammatory swelling due to several types of pierced earrings tend to show positive reactions to both gold and platinum, as well as nickel and palladium. The nickel allergy is known to be an important causative factor of atopic dermatitis (Klas et al., 1996). Therefore, care should be taken when using this material, as nickel allergies often cause serious allergic symptoms. In addition, one of the important results found in the current study was the positive reaction rate to palladium.

Due to the increase of patients with allergies noted over the last few years, practicing dentists need to have sufficient knowledge about dental metal allergies and be able to make these types of clinical diagnoses and then either treat these patients properly or refer them to specialists who can take over these treatment regimens. Current data indicate that practicing dentists need obtain further specialized knowledge about dental metal allergy in order to ensure the correct treatment of patients in their clinics.

8. Conclusion

All treatments that employ dental metal materials have the potential to cause allergic symptoms, and thus, proper preventive measures and treatment plans are required for these allergy patients. The results of our current research demonstrate the necessity for educating all dental practitioners in the recognition and treatment of dental metal allergy.

9. References

Akyol, A.,A. Boyvat,Y. Peksari & E. Gurgey (2005). Contact sensitivity to standard series allergens in 1038 patients with contact dermatitis in Turkey, *Contact Dermatitis* (52): 333-7.

Davies, R. J.,B. T. Butcher & J. E. Salvaggio (1977). Occupational asthma caused by low molecular weight chemical agents, *J Allergy Clin Immunol* (60): 93-5.

Davis, M. D.,K. Bhate,A. L. Rohlinger,S. A. Farmer,D. M. Richardson & A. L. Weaver (2008). Delayed patch test reading after 5 days: the Mayo Clinic experience, *J Am Acad Dermatol* (59): 225-33.

Fisher, A. A. (1973). *Contact Dermatitis,Second Ed.*, NY.

Fleischmann, P. (1928). Zur Frage der Gefährlichkeit Kleinster Quecksilbermengen, *Dtsch Med Wochen scher* (54): 304

Gawkrodger, D. J. (2005). Investigation of reactions to dental materials, *Br J Dermatol* (153): 479-85.

Geurtsen, W. (2002). Biocompatibility of dental casting alloys, *Crit Rev Oral Biol Med* (13): 71-84.

Groot, A. C. d. 2008. Patch Testing. Amsterdam: ELSEVIER.

Hamano, H.,K. Uoshima,W. P. Miao,T. Masuda,M. Matsumura,H. Hani,H. Kitazaki & M. Inoue (1998). [Investigation of metal allergy to constituent elements of intraoral restoration materials], *Kokubyo Gakkai Zasshi* (65): 93-9.

Hosoki, M.,E. Bando,K. Asaoka,H. Takeuchi & K. Nishigawa (2009). Assessment of allergic hypersensitivity to dental materials, *Biomed Mater Eng* (19): 53-61.

Hosoki, M.,E. Bando,M. Nakano,K. Nishigawa,K. Okura & Y. Yamazaki (2002). A clinical investigation for the patients with dental metal allergy, *Journal of Dental Research* (81): 412.

Hubler, W. R., Jr. & W. R. Hubler, Sr. (1983). Dermatitis from a chromium dental plate, *Contact Dermatitis* (9): 377-83.

Inoue, M. (1993). The Status Quo of Metal Allergy and Measures Against it in Dentistry, *J.Jpn.Prosthodont.Soc* (37): 1127-1138.

Ishii, N.,H. Ishii,H. Ono,Y. Horiuchi,H. Nakajima & I. Aoki (1990). Genetic control of nickel sulfate delayed-type hypersensitivity, *J Invest Dermatol* (94): 673-6.

Jean-Marie Lachapelle & H. I. Maibach (2009). *Patch Testing and Prick Testing: A Practical Guide Official Publication of ICDRG*, Springer, Heidelberg.

Jensen, C. S.,S. Lisby,O. Baadsgaard,A. Volund & T. Menne (2002). Decrease in nickel sensitization in a Danish schoolgirl population with ears pierced after implementation of a nickel-exposure regulation, *Br J Dermatol* (146): 636-42.

Khamaysi, Z.,R. Bergman & S. Weltfriend (2006). Positive patch test reactions to allergens of the dental series and the relation to the clinical presentations, *Contact Dermatitis* (55): 216-8.

Klas, P. A.,G. Corey,F. J. Storrs,S. C. Chan & J. M. Hanifin (1996). Allergic and irritant patch test reactions and atopic disease, *Contact Dermatitis* (34): 121-4.

Lam, W. S.,L. Y. Chan,S. C. Ho,L. Y. Chong,W. H. So & T. W. Wong (2008). A retrospective study of 2585 patients patch tested with the European standard series in Hong Kong (1995-99), *Int J Dermatol* (47): 128-33.

Larsson-Stymne, B. & L. Widstrom (1985). Ear piercing--a cause of nickel allergy in schoolgirls? , *Contact Dermatitis* (13): 289-93.

Lundstrom, I. M. (1984). Allergy and corrosion of dental materials in patients with oral lichen planus, *Int J Oral Surg* (13): 16-24.

Magnusson, B.,M. Bergman,B. Bergman & R. Soremark (1982). Nickel allergy and nickel-containing dental alloys, *Scand J Dent Res* (90): 163-7.

Minagi, S.,T. Sato,K. Suzuki & G. Nishigawa (1999). In situ microsampling technique for identification of elements of a restoration with exposed metal to identify potential allergens, *J Prosthet Dent* (82): 221-5.

Nakayama, H. (2002). New aspects of metal allergy, *Acta Dermatovenerol Croat* (10): 207-19.

Setcos, J. C.,A. Babaei-Mahani,L. D. Silvio,I. A. Mjor & N. H. Wilson (2006). The safety of nickel containing dental alloys, *Dent Mater* (22): 1163-8.

Shanon, J. (1965). Pseudo-atopic dermatitis. Contact dermatitis due to chrome sensitivity simulating atopic dermatitis, *Dermatologica* (131): 176-90.

Smith-Sivertsen, T.,L. K. Dotterud & E. Lund (1999). Nickel allergy and its relationship with local nickel pollution, ear piercing, and atopic dermatitis: a population-based study from Norway, *J Am Acad Dermatol* (40): 726-35.

Spiechowicz, E.,P. O. Glantz,T. Axell & P. Grochowski (1999). A long-term follow-up of allergy to nickel among fixed prostheses wearers, *Eur J Prosthodont Restor Dent* (7): 41-4.

Suzuki, N. (1995). Metal allergy in dentistry: detection of allergen metals with X-ray fluorescence spectroscope and its application toward allergen elimination, *Int J Prosthodont* (8): 351-9.

Uo, M. & F. Watari (2004). Rapid analysis of metallic dental restorations using X-ray scanning analytical microscopy, *Dent Mater* (20): 611-5.

Wataha, J. C. (2000). Biocompatibility of dental casting alloys: a review, *J Prosthet Dent* (83): 223-34.

Wiesenfeld, D.,M. M. Ferguson,A. Forsyth & D. G. MacDonald (1984). Allergy to dental gold, *Oral Surg Oral Med Oral Pathol* (57): 158-60.

Yanagi, T.,T. Shimizu,R. Abe & H. Shimizu (2005). Zinc dental fillings and palmoplantar pustulosis, *Lancet* (366): 1050.

Part 5

Contact Dermatitis in Children

7

Allergic Contact Dermatitis in Children

Alena Machovcová
University Hospital Motol, Prague
Czech Republic

1. Introduction

Contact allergy (CA), a pathologic response after (usually repeated) contact to environmental substances of low molecular weight occurring in a varying proportion of exposed persons, often results in clinical disease, allergic contact dermatitis (ACD), which can be disabling. CA is diagnosed by patch testing, a technique of controlled exposure of patients suspected to have ACD to a standardized set of substances frequently found to be the cause of ACD (Uter, 2004). ACD is an inflammatory reaction of the skin that follows percutaneous absorption of antigen from the skin surface and recruitment of previously sensitized, antigen-specific T lymphocytes into the skin (Rietschel & Fowler, 2001a). Although sensitivity to contact allergens occurs in 10-20% of the adult population, the exact incidence and prevalence of sensitization in children is unknown. ACD in children is not rare. The documented rates of ACD in children are on the increase (Militello et al., 2006; Goossens & Morren, 2006). Sensitization to contact allergens begins in infancy and continues to be more common in toddlers and young children. Infants, even neonates, may be sensitized (Fisher, 1994a; Bruckner et al., 2000). The rate of positive results may vary with referral patterns, selection criteria for patch testing, regional and social variations in allergens exposure and the allergen tested (Militello et al., 2006; Goossens & Morren, 2006; Wahlberg & Lindgerg, 2006).

2. Epidemiology (prevalence and incidence)

Previously, ACD was once wrongly considered uncommon in the pediatric population (Hjorth, 1981). It was thought that children had reduced exposure to contact allergens during childhood. The second reason was less susceptibility of the child immune system to contact allergens (Mortz & Andersen, 1999). However, during the last 10-20 years, several reports have described a considerable number of children with CA and ACD (Pevny et al., 1984a; Pevny et al., 1984b; Weston & Weston, 1984; Rademaker & Forsyth, 1989; Barros et al., 1991; Dotterund & Falk, 1995; Motolese et al., 1995; Katsarou et al., 1996; Rudzki & Rebandel, 1996; Stables et al., 1996; Manzini et al., 1998; Brasch & Geier, 1997), confirming that CA and ACD may be frequent in children and may cause significant problems. Prevalence of positive patch tests without clinical correlation (CA) in population-based studies is different from the prevalence of ACD (positive patch test with clinical correlation) in patients referred for patch testing.

2.1 Prevalence of contact allergy in a selected population

Patch test studies in series of selected children with suspected ACD have reported frequencies of positive reactions varying from 14% to 71% of patients. Of these, about 56-93% was of current relevance (Weston & Weston, 1984; Pevny et al., 1984b; Fisher, 1994a; Rudzki & Rebandel, 1996; Stables et al., 1996; Manzini et al., 1998; Bruckner et al., 2000; Machovcová et al., 2001; Wöhrl et al., 2003; Heine et al., 2004; Lewis et al., 2004; Jøhnke et al., 2004; Vozmediano & Hita, 2005; Wahlberg & Lindberg, 2006; Goossens & Morren, 2006; Jacob et al., 2008). Among the children with a positive patch test 3.2% to 54.4% had multiple contact allergies (Mortz & Andersen, 1999).

2.2 Prevalence of contact allergy in an unselected population

In the general pediatric population, the prevalence of ACD may be underestimated, which can be attributed to the low frequency of patch tests performed on children (compared to adults) and by the fact that in clinical practice, manifestations of ACD are often attributed to morphological look-alikes, such as atopic dermatitis (AD) or irritant dermatitis (Militello et al., 2006). The results from patch testing in children and adolescents in the general population revealed that 13-24.5% had positive patch tests to standard allergens. The prevalence of past or current relevant reactions was found to be 7%, with a higher risk seen in females (Dotterund & Falk, 1995; Bruckner et al., 2000; Mortz et al., 2001; Jacob et al., 2008). Few population-based studies have examined contact sensitization in asymptomatic healthy children. Barros et al. (Barros et al., 1991) patch tested 562 Portuguese school children (5-14 years old) with 25 allergens. Positive reactions were seen in 13.3%. Multiple sensitivities were seen in 2% of the children. Dotterud et Falk (Dotterund & Falk, 1995) patch tested 424 Norwegian school children (7-12 years old) with 20 allergens. One or more positive reactions were seen in 23.3%. Multiple sensitivities were seen in 8.5% of the children. Weston et al. (Weston et al., 1986) patch tested 314 otherwise healthy American children and adolescents under the age of 18 years with 20 allergens. He found at least one positive patch reaction in 20%. In Bruckner et al. (Bruckner et al., 2000) population-based study of 95 healthy asymptomatic children aged 6 to 67.5 months was showed that the prevalence of sensitization was 24.5% (≥ 1 positive reaction to an allergen). In our group of Czech schoolchildren, positive reactions were detected in 30.7%. Multiple sensitivities were seen in 8.7%. The relevance of reactions was 61% (Machovcová, 2006).

2.3 Prevalence related to sex

Sex may also play a role on the different prevalence in children. While some authors (Weston et al., 1986; Barros et al., 1991; Stables et al., 1996) detected similar prevalence in both boys and girls, other (Dotterund & Falk, 1995; Wantke et al., 1996; Goossens & Morren, 2006) reported a higher prevalence in girls. This is especially the case for nickel (Brasch & Geier, 1997; Wöhrl et al., 2003) and after the age of 12 (Rademaker & Forsyth, 1989; Rudzki & Rebandel, 1996; Katsarou et al., 1996; Goossens & Morren, 2006). Brasch & Geier (Brasch & Geier, 1997) found significantly more girls than boys reacted to nickel (25.0% vs. 4.5%). Hormonal factors may be a contributory factor here (Brasch & Geier, 1997; Goossens & Morren, 2006).

2.4 Prevalence related to age

Sensitization to contact allergens begins in infancy and continues to be more common in toddlers and young children (Seidenari et al., 1992; Giordano-Labadie et al., 1999; Vozmediano & Hita, 2005; Militello et al., 2006; Clayton et al., 2006; Garg et al., 2009; De Waard-van der Spek & Oranje, 2009), the age of sensitization can occur very early. In study of Bruckner et al. (Bruckner et al., 2000), 45% of patients with positive reactions were younger than 18 months. Even neonates may be sensitized (Fisher, 1994a; Bruckner et al., 2000). Fisher (Fisher, 1994a) reported a 1-week-old infant with strongly positive patch test reaction to epoxy resin, manifesting as band-like dermatitis above the wrist because of vinyl band that was made of an epoxy resin. A 7-month-old child has revealed ACD from nickel-plated snaps on the back (Fisher, 1994a). Motolese et al. (Motolese et al., 1995) studied 53 infants (3 months to 2 years) with dermatitis and patch tested them. Positive patch tests were seen in 32 (60%) and 20 out of the 32 sensitized infants had clinically relevant contact allergies. Hjorth (Hjorth, 1981) thought that patch test reactions in infants were predominantly irritant reactions, especially when testing with nickel sulfate. In a study of Jøhnke et al. (Jøhnke et al., 2004) it was confirmed that increasing numbers of infants positively patch tested to nickel sulfate but most reactions were transient and probably irritant or non-specific nature. Experimental CA to plants of the *Rhus* genus has also been induced in infants, showing that sensitization is possible (Epstein, 1961). Manzini et al. (Manzini et al., 1998) reported that the highest sensitization rate was noted in children aged up to 3 years. It is still unclear why some sensitivities, for example nickel, are prevalent in the young but less common in the old. Possible explanations include changing trends in exposure to nickel (i.e. increased use of imitation jewellery and different frequencies of ear piercing in different generations) or loss of clinical allergy because of avoidance, induction of tolerance, or inability to mount an immune response despite continuing exposure (Garg et al., 2009). Recall studies showed persistence of CA to nickel after 8 years in 79% and 60% to other allergens (Nielsen et al., 2001; Garg et al., 2009). Others found that lanolin, only 41% had persistent allergy at 5 years (Carmichael et al., 1991). The increase in fragrance allergy with age may be because of cumulative exposure to toiletries and increased use of medicaments (Garg et al., 2009).

3. Contact sensitisation and atopic dermatitis

The relationship between CA and atopy is frequently discussed and still not settled (Rystedt, 1985; Schnuch et al., 2006). Several studies have been performed in children with suspected CA or suffering from AD or chronic dermatitis. Patch testing in symptomatic children with dermatitis has revealed positive reactions in 15% to 52% of subjects (Rademaker & Forsyth, 1989; De Groot, 1990; Katsarou et al., 1996; Rudzki & Rebandel, 1996; Stables et al., 1996; Shah et al., 1997; Vozmediano & Hita, 2005; Goossens & Morren, 2006; Wahlberg & Lindgerg, 2006). Some authors have indicated that ACD is less prevalent in patients with AD (Uhr, 1960; Rystedt, 1985; De Groot, 1990; Katsarou et al., 1996; Stables et al., 1996; Brasch & Geier, 1997). Several authors were unable to detect differences between atopic and nonatopic subjects in this regard (Marghescu, 1985; Pambor et al., 1991; Goossens et al., 1995; Akhavan & Cohen, 2003; Beattie et al., 2007; Milingou et al., 2010). Against this others have even found a greater prevalence of ACD in patients with AD (De la Cuadra et al., 1990; Lammintausta et al., 1992; Dotterund & Falk, 1995; Lugovic & Lipozencic, 1997; Giordano-Labadie et al., 1999; Clayton et al., 2006). A higher prevalence of CA in AD could be explained by the alterations of the epidermal barrier and the greater permeability of irritated skin in AD that favours sensitization to ACD (Dotterund & Falk, 1995; Vozmediano & Hita, 2005). Moreover, patients with AD are chronically exposed to potentially more sensitizers because of the topical medications used for their skin (Giordano-Labadie et al., 1999; Vozmediano & Hita, 2005; Clayton et al., 2006). Also there exists a higher probability of false positive results in the patch tests conducted in patients with AD (Lammintausta et al., 1992; Mortz et al., 2001). Seguraro Rodriguez et al. (Segurado Rodriguez et al., 2004) found that a family history of AD (85%), female sex (74%) and age 11-16 (63%) were predisposing risk factors to sensitization. On the other hand, Giordano-Labadie et al. (Giordano-Labadie et al., 1999) systematically evaluated contact sensitization in a series of atopic pediatric patients. It was observed that 43% of the 114 children who patch tested had positive reactions without association with AD. From Vozmediano's (Vozmediano & Hita, 2005) point of view, AD did not affect the sensitization to the different allergens, although a higher number of irritative responses or false positives were frequently observed. Onder and Adisen reported only 0.3% of the patients having AD and positive patch test reactions in their study in a pediatric population in Turkey (Onder & Adisen, 2008).

4. Clinical presentation

The clinical characteristics of ACD are the same in children as in adults (Militello et al., 2006; Goossens & Morren, 2006). The classical clinical presentation of ACD is pruritic eczematous dermatitis. The location can be important for identification of the causal allergen since contact dermatitis is generally restricted to the contact site. Textile allergens usually cause dermatitis in areas in which the garment continually rubs against the skin, such as sub-axillary and/or flexural areas of the extremities. Cosmetic allergens tend to produce facial, neck or periorbital dermatitis. Shoe allergens often present on the dorsum of the feet (Goossens, 2001; Militello et al., 2006; Goossens & Morren, 2006). Spreading of the dermatitis, often in the form of small papules, may occur far from the original contact site and may be generalized. This can be explained by hematogenous dissemination of the allergens (Goossens, 2001) or by contact with allergenic or allergen-contaminated surfaces, transfer of an allergen via the hands to the face or other sites, which gives rise to an 'ectopic' contact dermatitis. CA can be caused also by products that have come in contact with the parents or other persons in the environment of the children ('connubial' or 'consort' dermatitis). The 'ectopic' or 'connubial' reactions are commonly involved the skin of the eyelids or neck. Additionally, distant or widespread eruptions (commonly referred to as 'Id' reactions) can often be triggered by localized ACD to such chemicals as nickel and poison ivy (Goossens, 2001; Militello et al., 2006; Goossens & Morren, 2006). Untreated reactions from highly potent allergens, such a poison ivy, can be severe and last for several weeks (Militello et al., 2006). Continued exposure even to low levels of allergen can perpetuate these skin eruptions indefinitely. Recognizing potential pediatric patients with ACD either as the primary diagnosis or the confounding factor is crucial. Often the findings are difficult to distinguish, clinically and histopathologically, from AD or irritant dermatitis (Goossens, 2001; Militello et al., 2006; Goossens & Morren, 2006).

5. Diagnosis and patch testing in children

Diagnosis rests on taking a substantial clinical history. Essential is an extensive and standardized anamnesis that covers all possible etiological factors like hobbies, leisure time activities, use of topical pharmaceutical products and cosmetics and contact with plants (Goossens, 2001). The children and their parents can themselves provide many indications but often need to be convinced that the allergenic product may not have been introduced only recently into their environment. Indeed, it can take several days before the clinical symptoms and signs appear after the contact. The delay in reaction by 24-48 hours after allergen exposure can make difficulties to establish (Goossens, 2001). Children and their parents are not typically aware of this delay in reaction and often search for immediate associations. A detailed history of events during the week preceding the onset of symptoms is vital (Militello et al., 2006).

The gold standard for definitive diagnosis of ACD is epicutaneous patch testing (Militello et al., 2006; Goossens & Morren, 2006). Most authors agree that the patch testing in children is safe (Weston et al., 1989; Rademaker & Forsyth, 1989; Fisher, 1994b; Goossens & Morren, 2006), the only problems being mainly technical due to small patch test surface (Rademaker & Forsyth, 1989; Goossens & Morren, 2006), hypermobility, particularly in smaller children (Shah et al., 1997; Goossens & Morren, 2006). Patch testing involves the placement of a small amount of potential allergens under occlusion on the patient's back. These patches are typically removed after 48 hours and an initial reading is performed. A delayed reading at 72 and/or at 96 hours is recommended. Positive reactions are evaluated according to the criteria of the International Contact Dermatitis Research Group as – (negative), +- (doubtful) and +, ++, +++ (weak, moderate and strong reaction, respectively) depending on the grade of erythema, induration or blistering that occurs at the site of allergen placement (Wahlberg & Lindgerg, 2006). The patch test concentrations have been discussed in detail in the literature (Goossens & Morren, 2006). Some authors have recommended lower concentrations (Hjorth, 1981; Pambor et al., 1991), particularly with regard to specific allergens such as nickel and formaldehyde (Fisher, 1991), mercurials (Fisher, 1994b), potassium dichromate and thiuram mix (Fisher, 1994b). The others use the same test concentrations as those used in adults (Pevny et al., 1984a; Pevny et al., 1984b; Stables et al., 1996; Seidenari et al., 1992; Motolese et al., 1995; Worm et al., 2007).

Children should be tested strictly based on the indication using a standard protocol. A negative patch test result does not exclude contact dermatitis. False-negative reactions have various causes, often 'missed' allergen, which may be picked up by detailed questioning (Goossens, 2001; Goossens & Morren, 2006). For the skin tests, the possible risks of overlooking a CA are thus centred on the allergen itself, the test method, the test concentration and vehicle used, the time of reading and, finally, the relevance (Goossens, 2001).

6. Clinical relevance

Contact sensitization, however, does not necessarily equate with clinical diseases. Clinical relevance of allergic reactions on patch testing was determined according to the clinical history, type of dermatitis and the allergen concerned. Relevance of allergens should be determined for all patients with one or more positive reactions. Clinical relevance was confirmed if the allergen was found to be present in the patient's environment, the dermatitis corresponded to point(s) of contact with the allergen and the dermatitis significantly improved upon isolation of the allergen, or recurred with re-challenge (positive use test) (Jacob et al., 2008). Reported clinical relevance in children has been varied between 20% and 93% (Pevny et al., 1984b; Rademaker & Forsyth, 1989; Pambor et al., 1991; Stables, 1996; Mortz & Andersen, 1999).

7. The common allergens in children

Nickel is always the most common allergen in children, followed by cobalt, mercurials (thimerosal and metallic mercury), rubber chemicals (thiuram mix, carba mix, mercapto mix and mercaptobenzothiazole, PPD) and fragrance mix. The most frequent sources are costume jewellery (nickel in earrings), medications, footwear, cosmetics and plants (Rademaker & Forsyth, 1989; Barros et al., 1991; Stables et al., 1996; Militello et al., 2006; Goossens & Morren, 2006).

7.1 Nickel

Nickel is by far the most common allergen in patients of all ages, including children. Nickel was the top allergen in children in 14 of the 17 studies of patch testing summarized by Mortz and Andersen (Mortz & Andersen, 1999). Even in younger children nickel allergy is not uncommon (Jøhnke et al., 2004). Published rates of nickel sensitization in children range between 10% and 24% (Wöhrl et al., 2003; Heine et al., 2004; Lewis et al., 2004; Seidenari et al., 2005; Vozmediano & Hita, 2005; Clayton et al., 2006; Militello et al., 2006; Goossens & Morren, 2006; Milingou et al., 2010). Ear piercing along with atopy is regarded as a major risk factor for the development of nickel sensitization, especially in girls (Militello et al., 2006; Goossens & Morren, 2006). Nickel sensitization sources in children are numerous: jewellery (earrings), jean studs, belt buckles, zippers or buttons (Clayton et al., 2006). Sensitization to nickel is not necessarily followed by ACD, but infants with a reproducible positive reaction to nickel sulfate could represent a group at risk of developing clinically manifest nickel dermatitis later in life (Magnusson & Moller, 1979). In agreement with earlier studies in older children and adults (Dotterund & Falk, 1995; Mortz et al., 2001; Uter et al., 2004; Jøhnke et al., 2004), a female predominance of positive reactions to nickel sulfate was found in infants (girls 13.1% and boys 4.0%). Despite a marked decrease in nickel allergy and nickel dermatitis in young women after nickel regulation came into force (Schnuch & Uter, 2003; Thyssen et al., 2009; 2011), the prevalence of nickel allergy remains very high, and seems to have stabilized at a high level (Schnuch et al., 2011). However, women who were ear-pierced after regulatory intervention in Denmark had a significantly lower prevalence of nickel allergy and dermatitis than women who were ear-pierced before (Thyssen et al., 2009; 2011). It is important to emphasize that nickel allergy remains very prevalent in some European countries. The proportion of positive patch test reactions to nickel sulfate has remained stable at 10%-20% among young female German dermatitis patients (< 18 years) since the beginning of the new millennium (Schnuch et al., 2011). The 2005-2006 clinical patch test data registered in 10 European countries and reported to the European Surveillance System on Contact Allergies revealed high prevalence of nickel allergy in western, southern, central and north-eastern Europe, being, respectively, 20.8%, 24.5%, 19.7% and 22.4% (Uter et al., 2009). There may be several explanations for this finding (Thyssen et al., 2011), but it is generally accepted that excessive nickel release from consumer items is one of the most important single factors (Schnuch & Uter, 2003).

7.2 Thiomersal and metallic mercury

Sensitization to thiomersal (an organic mercurial compound) is frequently observed in infants and children. The widespread use as a preservative in a variety of compounds, including vaccine and antitoxin preparations, ophthalmic drops and contact lens solutions, may explain the high rate of positive patch test reactions (Katsarou et al., 1996; Militello et al., 2006; Goossens & Morren, 2006; Milingou et al., 2010). Low clinical relevance along with sensitization rates is probably related to its presence in vaccines (Novák et al., 1986; Osawa et al., 1991; Lee et al., 2009). Recently, percentages of sensitization in children have increased from 2.3% (Barros et al., 1991) to 10% (Möller, 1997) due to iatrogenic sources (antiseptics, topical medications, thermometers and vaccines) and footwear (Novák et al., 1986; Osawa et al., 1991; Militello et al., 2006; Goossens & Morren, 2006; Lee et al., 2009).

7.3 Topical antibiotics

Neomycin, bacitracin and gentamycin are topical antibiotics with high rates of allergic contact sensitization in children (Heine et al., 2004; Seidenari et al., 2005; Jacob et al. 2008). Neomycin sulfate has remained second place in the most common culprits in ACD for close to 25 years (Spann et al., 2003; Lee et al., 2009). It is a topical antibiotic with multiple clinical indications, including use for superficial wounds or burns and can be found in many over-the-counter products in the US or Europe. It is also formulated in combinations with other antibiotics, antifungals or corticosteroids (Lee et al., 2009). Menezes de Pádua et al. (Menezes de Pádua et al., 2005) found 2.5% positive reactions to neomycin, while in 1.1%, ACD was additionally diagnosed.

7.4 Cosmetics allergens

The market for cosmetic products specially formulated for children is expanding and usage of cosmetics being seen to increase in children. Consequently, one can expect cosmetics to become more important causes of ACD in children (Goossens et al., 2002). At least one cosmetic or cosmetic ingredient gave a positive reaction in 30% of the children investigated (Goossens et al., 2002; Goossens & Morren, 2006). Almost every ingredient may be responsible for cosmetic dermatitis (Goossens et al., 2002; Goossens & Morren, 2006). Fisher (Fisher, 1995) further stated that children often become allergic to cosmetics used by the mother or the person taking care of them. The localizations often involved seem to be the forehead and the cheeks, with perfume, lipstick, hairspray or nail lacquer as the responsible agents (Fisher 1995; Goossens et al., 2002; Buckley et al., 2003; Goossens & Morren, 2006). However, children often use cosmetic products themselves and this may not always be revealed immediately (Goossens et al., 2002; Goossens & Morren, 2006).

7.4.1 Fragrances

The use of cosmetic products in babies and young children can cause perfume allergy (Fisher 1995; Goossens et al., 2002; Buckley et al., 2003; Goossens & Morren, 2006). A large numbers of perfumed products are marketed especially for children (Rastogi et al., 1999; Kohl et al., 2002). Fragrance allergy is increasingly common and even young children are exposed (Rastogi et al., 1999). Exposure is usually due to perfumes or to other aromatic topical products such as moisturizers or deodorants. Typical sites of involvement include face, neck and axillae, in addition to full systemic contact dermatitis (Tomar et al., 2005; Garg et al., 2009; Lee et al., 2009). Fragrance allergy is usually detected by patch testing to three mixtures of scented compounds: Fragrance Mix I, Fragrance Mix II and *Myroxylon pereirae* tree extract (Balsam of Peru). The rate of sensitization to fragrance appears to increase with age (Buckley et al., 2003; Lee et al., 2009). The *Myroxylon pereirae* tree extract

(Balsam of Peru) is used as a screen for fragrance allergy, due to its wide usage and natural cross-reactivity with other frequently encountered fragrances (Tomar et al., 2005; Garg et al., 2009; Lee et al., 2009). These allergens (or chemically similar ones) are also used in soft drinks and flavouring such as cinnamon, cloves, curry and vanilla. Although dietary intervention remains controversial, there is evidence that it may help those with significant disease that is not resolving with more typical fragrance avoidance (Magnusson & Wilkinson, 1975; Salam & Fowler Jr., 2001; Tomar et al., 2005). Although guidelines for the maximum concentration of preservatives and fragrances in cosmetics have been provided (Goossens et al., 2004), it has been demonstrated that toys may contain much higher concentrations of fragrance (Rastogi et al., 1999). No extra safety requirements for toys intended for children are required (White, 2000).

7.4.2 Preservatives

Conti et al. (Conti et al., 1997) reviewed contact sensitization to 8 preservatives (imiadazolidinyl urea, diazolidinyl urea, parabens, formaldehyde, quaternium-15, Katon CG, Euxyl K400 and butylated hydroxyanizole) in the child population and found 7.3% of the children reacted positively. Almost 50% of preservative-sensitive children had AD. Baby toilet tissues have been occasionally reported to cause CA in babies and those who take care of them. The allergens considered most often are fragrances and preservatives. Methylchloroisothiazolinone and methylisothiazolinone (MCI/MI) is widely used as a preservative in many products (De Groot & Herxheimer, 1989). Tosti et al. (Tosti et al., 2003) found MCI/MI to be a frequent cause of ACD, i.e. in 7 of 95 children between 3 and 11 years old were positive to MCI/MI. The use of moist toilet papers (baby wipes) can be responsible for ACD, especially of perianal area (De Groot et al., 1991). MCI/MI was replaced from them by other preservatives, particularly with Euxyl K400 (methydibromoglutaronitrile and phenoxyethanol) (Senff et al., 1989) and 1,2-dibromo-2,4-dicyanobutane (Van Ginkel & Rutdervoort, 1995).

7.4.3 Sorbitan sesquioleate

De Waard-van der Spek and Oranje (De Waard-van der Spek & Oranje, 2009) found 3 children patch tested positive to sorbitan sesquioleate (SSO), all clinically relevant. Two children used emollient contained SSO as emulsifier. They also reported a child positive patch tested to Adaptic non-adhering dressing containing SSO. Castanedo-Tardan and Jacob (Castanedo-Tardan & Jacob, 2008) reported the case series of 6 pediatric patients with clinically relevant contact allergy to SSO. 5 children were atopics and suffered with recalcitrant dermatitis.

7.5 *Para*-Phenylenediamine and tattoos

An increased prevalence of *para*-Phenylenediamine (PPD) allergy has been noted in the pediatric population. Eczematous reactions are mostly seen at the site of the tattoo and they may be long-lasting (Lewis et al., 2004). Henna dye is a dark green powder, used for hair dyeing and body tattooing. Henna itself is relatively safe. However, PPD is added on an illegal basis in semi-permanent tattoos (black henna tattoos), in order to obtain a darker colour and a faster drying time than natural henna can provide. Although many parents and consumers believe these black henna tattoos to be temporary, adverse events to them (scaring and sensitization) can be permanent. PPD is a very potent contact sensitizer included in the European baseline series for patch testing. PPD is also contained in permanent hair dyes and related compounds (Lee et al., 2009). The content of PPD in semi-permanent tattoo ink has been reported to vary between 0.4 and 15.7%, far exceeding the limit permissible for hair dyes (<6%) (Brancaccio et al., 2002; Avnstorp et al., 2002; Sosted et al., 2006; Lee et al., 2009). The long duration of skin contact, the high concentrations of sensitizing materials (diaminobenzenes or diaminotoluenes) and the lack of a neutralizing agent increase the risk of skin sensitization. Because of the worldwide vogue for skin painting, a greater number of patients sensitized to PPD and diaminobenzenes or diaminotoluenes can be expected (Le Coz et al., 2000; Onder et al., 2001; Neri et al., 2002; Jovanovic & Slavkovic-Jovanovic, 2009). The unusually severe reactions to PPD in young 12 to 15 year old adolescents have occurred after dyeing their hair having been previously sensitized to PPD in black henna tattoo at a younger age. In some cases, the children developed severe angioedema-like reactions necessitating admission to hospital and intensive care treatment (Sosted et al., 2006). Severe allergic reactions were reported in 1.4% of women and 1.3% of men after dying their hair (Sosted et al., 2005). Sensitization to PPD is potential for lifelong sensitization and systemic contact dermatitis can be evoked with exposure to cross-reactors such as benzocaine, diuretics (hydrochlorothiazide) and sulfonamide medications (Sosted et al., 2006; Lee et al., 2009). Notably, 25% of those allergic to PPD can also be reactive to semi-permanent dyes found in synthetic clothing. PPD base, being a part of the European baseline series, is regarded as a screening agent for contact allergy to *para* and azo compounds in hair dyes, but not for textile and leather dye allergy (Koopmans & Bruynzeel, 2003).

7.6 Rubber compounds

Rubber additives are typically present in many rubber products (e.g. elastic waistbands, socks, swimwear, shoes, toys, cosmetic applicators and adhesives) and could be main allergens from them. Thiurams, mercapto chemicals and less commonly carbamates are the responsible allergens in rubber allergy in children; thiourea derivates in neoprene may also be the cause of dermatitis (Goossens & Morren, 2006; Lee et al., 2009). Roul et al. (Roul et al., 1998) reported a particular type of diaper dermatitis called 'Lucky Luke' dermatitis. The rubber parts used for a new anti-leaking system in these diapers provoked the reaction. Mercaptobenzothiazole and thiuram derivates are also present in certain types of glues (Roul et al., 1996; Cockayne et al., 1998). Type I allergic reactions may also occur (contact urticaria syndrome), sometimes associated with a type IV reaction. It is typical for children who had undergone multiple surgical operations (for example children suffering from spina bifida). Moreover, these children are particularly susceptible to natural rubber latex proteins in this regard (Goossens & Morren, 2006).

7.7 Toxicodendron dermatitis (Poison Ivy, Poison Oak, Poison Sumac)

Toxicodendron (Poison Ivy) dermatitis can occur at any age, although infants are apparently not as easily sensitized as adults. After the age of 3, children become highly susceptible and by 12 years of age nearly all have become sensitized to poison ivy (Kligman 1974). Plants belonging to the Rhus family are the ones most often involved in ACD among children living in the United States (Goossens & Morren, 2006). The oleoresin (urushiol) of the sap of the *Toxicodendron* plants contains catechols, which are very strong sensitizing chemicals. The eruption produced by poison ivy is characterized by redness, papules, vesicles and bullae plus linear streaking. Occasionally, urticaria and eruptions, resembling erythema multiforme, measles or scarlatina, occur from systemic absorption of the poison ivy antigen (Rietschel & Fowler Jr., 2008b). Exposure can be direct or indirect, such as transfers of the allergen via animals, tools, clothing, golf clubs, etc. (Goossens & Morren, 2006; Rietschel & Fowler Jr., 2008b), which is more difficult to diagnose (Epstein 1971). A few cases of phytophotodermatitis from *Toxicodendron* in children were also reported (Goossens & Morren, 2006).

8. Treatment

The cornerstone of treatment of ACD is proper allergen avoidance. Once an allergen is identified, patients must be educated on potential exposures, cross-reacting chemicals, preventive measures, as well as offered suggestions for avoidance. This may be especially difficult in households with small children affected, as the products that are used by the patents and sibling may also need to be considered as sources for allergen exposures.

Emollients can be added after a bath in an effort to retain hydration and restore the barrier function of the skin. Barrier repair also decreases pruritus and reduces visible scaling and dryness. Physical barrier creams may be useful in cases in which the allergen exposure cannot be avoided. Patients should apply the creams before and during the exposure in an effort to decrease absorption (Lee et al., 2009).

Topical corticosteroids are the first-line treatment modality for mild cases of ACD but they are not without risk and can cause multiple cutaneous side effects with extensive and long term use (Militello et al., 2006; Goossens & Morren, 2006; Jacob & Castanedo-Tardan, 2007; Lee et al., 2009). When selecting a topical corticosteroid for treatment, it is important to choose one that the patient is not allergic to in terms of the active ingredient (the steroid component) and inactive ingredients in the vehicle (Lee et al., 2009). As with any topical steroid, the risk of atrophy, teleangiectasias, tachyphylaxis and systemic absorption should be kept in mind, especially in areas of increased sensitivity such as face, groin and flexural area (Militello et al., 2006).

Topical calcineurin inhibitors (TCIs) are another therapeutic option and should be considered when steroid-sparing agents are required. These agents can be used for certain areas, such as the face, axilla and groin, which are more susceptible to steroid-induced atrophy (Lee et al., 2009).

In cases of widespread and severe reactions, Militello et al. (Militello et al., 2006) recommended at least 3 weeks of oral prednisone in combination with topical therapy. Shorter courses often lead to rebound flares of the dermatitis. Systemic corticosteroids are generally started at 1 mg/kg per day (Brasch, 2009). Oral H1-antihistamines are widely used as an adjuvant nonspecific treatment for pruritus in infants and children. They also cause drowsiness that may help with sleeping disturbances from pruritus (Militello et al., 2006; Lee et al., 2009).

9. Conclusions

ACD in infancy is more frequent than was initially suggested, although its true prevalence and incidence continue to be unknown. Age and sex influence its development, but the principal factor associated with ACD is the pattern of exposure to the various allergens (Vozmediano & Hita, 2005). In the unselected population, the prevalence of CA is about 20% (Mortz & Andersen, 1999; Weston & Weston, 1984; Barros et al., 1991), while in the selected population, the prevalence of ACD is found to be variable, with a mean of 40% (Mortz & Andersen, 1999; Wöhrl et al., 2003; Heine et al., 2004; Lewis et al., 2004; Seidenari et al., 2005; Vozmediano & Hita, 2005; Militello et al., 2006; Goossens & Morren, 2006; Jacob et al., 2008). The susceptibility to contact sensitization increases with the age. The most important allergens observed in this population are metals, mercury, pharmaceutical products and cosmetics (Vozmediano & Hita, 2005; Militello et al., 2006; Goossens & Morren, 2006; Jacob et al., 2008). ACD in childhood may also affect decisions regarding future occupations in adulthood. Therefore, it is very important that any CA in a child is recognized and dealt with in time. The impact of CA must not be underestimated, both on a complex individual scale of quality of life and socio-economically, for example, due to job options (Uter et al., 2004). Patch testing is both well tolerated and diagnostically essential in the evaluation of pediatric patients with potential ACD. Once allergen is documented, treatment relies on symptomatic use of topical or oral corticosteroids and meticulous allergen avoidance (Militello et al., 2006). Good information on preventing the development of ACD in children is useful for the caregivers.

10. Acknowledgment

Many thanks to Mrs. Susan Harley and Mr. Christopher J. Garlick for their linguistic assistance.

The project was supported by grants MZOFNM 2005/6904

11. References

Akhavan, A. & Cohen, SR. (2003). The relationship between atopic dermatitis and contact dermatitis. *Clin Dermatol* 21(2): 158-162.

Avnstorp, C., Rastogi, SC. & Menné, T. (2002). Acute fingertip dermatitis from temporary tattoo and quantitative chemical analysis of the product. *Contact Dermatitis* 47: 119-120.

Barros, MA., Baptista, A., Correia, TM. & Azevedo, F. (1991). Patch testing in children: a study of 562 schoolchildren. *Contact Dermatitis* 25: 156–159.

Beattie, PE., Green, C., Lowe, G. & Lewis-Jones, MS. (2007). Which children should we patch test? *Clin Exp Dermatol* 32: 6-11.

Brancaccio, RR., Brown, LH., Chang, YT., Fogelman, JP., Mafong, EA. & Cohen, DE. (2002). Identification and quantification of para-phenylenediamine in a temporary black henna tattoo. *Am J Contact Dermat* 13: 15-18.

Brasch, J. & Geier, J. (1997). Patch test results in schoolchildren. *Contact Dermatitis* 37: 286-293.

Brasch J. (2009). Contact Allergy in children. *Hautarzt* 60: 194-196.

Bruckner, AL., Weston, WL. & Morelli, JG. (2000). Does sensitization to contact allergens begin in infancy? *Pediatrics* 105: 3-9.

Buckley, DA., Rycroft, RJG., White, IR. & McFadden, JP. (2003). The frequency of fragrance allergy in patch-tested patients increases with age. *Br J Dermatol* 149: 986-989.

Carmichael, AJ., Foulds, IS. & Bransbury, DS. (1991). Loss of lanolin patch-test positivity. *Br J Dermatol* 125: 573-576.

Castanedo-Tardan, MP. & Jacob, SE. (2008). Allergic contact dermatitis to sorbitan sesquioleate in children. *Contact Dermatitis* 58: 171-171.

Clayton, TH., Wilkinson, SM., Rawcliffe, C., Pollock, B. & Clark, SM. (2006). Allergic contact dermatitis in children: should pattern of dermatitis determinate referral? A retrospective study of 500 children tested between 1995 and 2004 in one U.K. centre. *Br J Dermatol* 154: 114-117.

Cockayne, SE., Shah, M., Messenger, AG. & Gawkrodger, DJ. (1998). Foot dermatitis in children: causative allergens and follow-up. *Contact Dermatitis* 38: 203-206.

Conti, A., Motolese, A., Manzini, BM. & Seidenari, S. (1997). Contact sensitisation to preservatives in children. *Contact Dermatitis* 37: 35-36.

De Groot, AC. & Herxheimer, A. (1989). Isothiazolinone preservative: cause of a continuing epidemic cosmetic dermatitis. *Lancet* 1: 314-316.

De Groot, AC. (1990). The frequency of contact allergy in atopic patients with dermatitis. *Contact Dermatitis* 22: 273-277.

De Groot, AC., Baar, TJ., Terpstra, H. & Weyland, JW. (1991). Contact allergy to moist toilet paper. *Contact Dermatitis* 24: 135-136.

De la Cuadra, J., Sanz, J. & Martorell, A. (1990). Prevalence of positive epicutaneous tests in atopic and non-atopic children without dermatitis. *Contact Dermatitis* 23: 242-243.

De Waard-van der Spek, FB. & Oranje, AP. (2009). Patch Test in Children with Suspected Allergic Contact Dermatitis: A Prospective Study and Review of the Literature. *Dermatology* 218: 119-125.

Dotterund, LK. & Falk, ES. (1995). Contact allergy in relation to hand eczema and atopic diseases in north Norwergian schoolchildren. *Acta Paediatr* 84: 402-406.

Epstein, WL. (1961). Contact-type delayed hypersensitivity in infants and children: introduction of rhus sensitivity. *Pediatrics* 27: 51-53.

Fisher, AA. (1991). Nickel dermatitis in children. *Cutis* 47: 19-21.

Fisher, AA. (1994). Allergic contact dermatitis in early infancy. *Cutis* 54: 300-302a.

Fisher, AA. (1994). Patch testing in children including early infancy. *Cutis* 54: 387-388b.

Fisher, AA. (1995). Cosmetic dermatitis in childhood. *Cutis* 55: 15-16.

Garg, S., McDonagh, AJG. & Gawkroder, DJ. (2009). Age- and sex-related variations in allergic contact dermatitis to common allergens. *Contact Dermatitis* 61: 46-47.

Giordano-Labadie, F., Rancé, F., Pellegrin, F., Bazex, J., Dutau, G. & Schwarze, HP. (1999). Frequency of contact allergy in children with atopic dermatitis: results of a prospective study of 137 cases. *Contact Dermatitis* 40: 192–195.

Goossens, A., Motolese, A., Manzini, BM. & Donini, M. (1995). Patch testing in infants. *Am J Contact Dermat* 6: 153-156.

Goossens, A. (2001). Minimizing the Risks of Missing a Contact Allergy. *Dermatology* 202: 186-189.

Goossens, A., Kohl, L., Blondeel, A. & Song, M. (2002). Allergic contact dermatitis from cosmetics. Retrospective analysis of 819 patch-tested patients. *Dermatology* 204: 334-337.

Goossens, A., Kütting, B., Brehler, R. & Traupe, H. (2004). Alergic contact dermatitis in children – strategies of prevention and risk management. *Eur J Dermatol* 14: 80-85.

Goossens, A. & Morren, M. (2006). Contact Allergy in Children, In: Frosch PJ, Menne T, Lepoittevin J-P (Eds.), *Contact Dermatitis,* 4th ed., Springer-Verlag, Berlin, pp. 811-830.

Hjorth, N. (1981) Contact dermatitis in children. *Acta Derm Venerol (Stockh)* 95: 36-39.

Heine, G., Schnuch, A., Uter, W. & Worm, M. (2004). Frequency of contact allergy in German children and adolescents patch tested between 1995 and 2002: results from Information Network of Departments and the German Contact Dermatitis Research Group. *Contact Dermatitis* 51: 111-117.

Jacob, SE., Brod, B. & Crawford, GH. (2008). Clinically Relevant Patch Test Reactions in Children - A United States Based Study. *Pediatr Dermatol* 25: 520-527.

Jacob, SE. & Castanedo-Tardan, MP. (2007). Pharmacotherapy for allergic contact dermatitis. *Expert Opin Pharmacother* 8: 2757-2774.

Jøhnke, H., Norberg, LA., Vach, W., Bindslev-Jensen, C., Høst, A. & Andersen, KE. (2004). Reactivity to patch tests with nickel sulfate and fragrance in infants. *Contact Dermatitis* 51: 141-147.

Jovanovic, DL. & Slavkovic-Jovanovic, MR. (2009). Allergic contact dermatitis from temporary henna tattoo. *J Dermatol* 36: 63-65.

Katsarou, A., Koufou, V., Armenaka, M., Kalogeromitros, D., Papanayotou, G. & Vareltzidis, A. (1996). Patch tests in children: a review of 14 years' experience. *Contact Dermatitis* 34: 70-71.

Kligman, AM. (1974). Poison ivy *(Rhus)* dermatitis. *Arch Dermatol* 90: 535.

Kohl, L., Blondeel, A. & Song, M. (2002). Allergic contact dermatitis from cosmetics. Retrospective analysis of 819 patch-tested patients. *Dermatology* 204: 334-337.

Koopmans, AK. & Bruynzeel, DP. (2003). Is PPD a useful screening agent? *Contact Dermatitis* 48: 89-92.

Lammintausta, K., Kalimo, K. & Fagerlund, VL. (1992). Patch test reactions in atopic patients. *Contact Dermatitis* 26: 234-240.

Le Coz, CJ., Lefebvre, C., Keller, F. & Grosshans, E. (2000). Allergic Contact Dermatitis Caused by Skin Painting (Pseudotattooing) With Black Henna, a Mixture of Henna and p-Phenylenediamine and Its Derivates. *Arch Dermatol* 136: 1515-1517.

Lee, PW., Elsaie, ML. & Jacob, SE. (2009). Allergic contact dermatitis in children: common allergens and treatment: a review. *Curr Opin Pediatr* 21: 491-498.

Lewis, VJ., Stathmam, BN. & Chowdhury, MMU. (2004). Allergic contact dermatitis in 191 consecutively patch tested children. *Contact Dermatitis* 51: 155-156.

Lugovic, L. & Lipozencic, J. (1997). Contact hypersensitivity in atopic dermatitis. *Arh Hig Rada Toksikol* 48: 287-296.

Machovcová, A., Čapková, Š., Konkol'ová, R. & Hercogová, J. (2001). První výsledky epikutánních testů u dětí s atopickou dermatitidou. *Alergie* 1: 9-13.

Machovcová A. (2006). Frequency of Contact Allergy in Children and Adolescents in Czech Republic, *Proceedings of 15th EADV Congress From Hippocrates to Modern Dermatology,* Medimond, Rhodes (Greese), pp. 837-840.

Manzini, BM., Ferdani, G., Simonetti, V., Donini, M. & Seidenari, S. (1998). Contact sensitization in children. *Pediatr Dermatol* 15: 12-17.

Magnusson, B. & Wilkinson, DS (1975). Cinnamic aldehyde in toothpaste. Clinical aspects and patch tests. *Contact Dermatitis* 1: 70-76.

Magnusson, B. & Moller, H. (1979). Contact allergy without skin disease. *Acta Derm Venereol Suppl (Stockh)* 59: 113-115.

Marghescu, S. (1985). Patch test reactions in atopic patients. *Acta Derm Venereol (Stockh)* 114(Suppl.): 113-116.

Menezes de Pádua, CA., Schnuch, A., Lessmann, H., Geier, J., Pfahlberg, A. & Uter, W. (2005). Contact Allergy to neomycin sulfate: results of a multifactorial analysis. *Pharmacoepidemiol Drug Saf* 14: 725-733.

Milingou, M., Tagka, A., Armenaka, M., Kimpouri, K., Kouimintzis, D. & Katsarou, A. (2010). Patch tests in children: a review of 13 years of experience in comparison with previous data. *Pediatr Dermatol* 27: 255-259.

Militello, G., Jacob, SE. & Crawford, GH. (2006). Allergic contact dermatitis in children. *Curr Opin Pediatr* 18: 385-390.

Möller, H. (1997). Merthiolate allergy: a nation-wide iatrogenic sensitisation. *Acta Derm Venereol* 50: 509-517.

Mortz, CG. & Andersen, KE. (1999). Allergic contact dermatitis in children and adolescents. *Contact Dermatitis* 41: 121-30.

Mortz, CG., Lauritsen, JM., Bindslev-Jensen, C. & Andersen, KE. (2001). Prevalence of atopic dermatitis, asthma, allergic rhinitis, and hand and contact dermatitis in adolescents. The Odense Adolescence Cohort Study on Atopic Diseases and Dermatitis. *Br J Dermatol* 144: 523-532.

Motolese, A., Manzini, BM. & Donini, M. (1995). Patch tests in infants. *Am J Contact Dermatol* 6: 153-156.

Neri, I., Guareshi, E., Savoia, F. & Patrizi, A. (2002). Childhood allergic contact dermatitis from henna tattoo. *Pediatr Dermatol* 19: 503-505.

Nielsen, NH., Linneberg, A., Menné T., Madsen F., Frølund L., Dirksen A. & Jørgensen T. (2001). Persistence of contact allergy among Danish adults: an 8-year follow-up study. *Contact Dermatitis* 45: 350-353.

Novák, M., Kvíčalová, E. & Friedländerová, B. (1986). Reactions to merthiolate in infants. *Contact Dermatitis* 15: 309-310.

Onder, M., Atahan, CA., Oztas, P. & Oztas, MO. (2001). Temporary henna tattoo reactions in children. *Int J Dermatol* 40: 577-579.

Onder, M. & Adisen, E. (2008). Patch test results in a Turkish paediatric population. *Contact Dermatitis* 58: 63-65.

Osawa, J., Kitamura, K. & Ikezawa, Z. (1991). A probable role for vaccines containing thimerosal in thimerosal hypersensitivity. *Contact Dermatitis* 24: 178-182.

Pambor, M., Winkler, S. & Bloch, Y. (1991). Allergic contact dermatitis in children. *Contact Dermatitis* 24: 72-74.

Pevny, I., Brennenstuhl, M. & Razinskas, G. (1984). Patch testing in children (I). Collective test results; skin testability in children. *Contact Dermatitis* 11: 201-206.

Pevny, I., Brennenstuhl, M. & Razinskas, G. (1984). Patch testing in children (II). Results and case reports. *Contact Dermatitis* 11: 302-310.

Rademaker, M. & Forsyth, A. (1989). Contact dermatitis in children. *Contact Dermatitis* 20: 104-107.

Rastogi, SC., Johansen, JD., Menné, T., Frosch, P., Bruze, M., Andersen, KE., Lepoittevin, JP., Wakelin, S. & White, IR. (1999). Contents of fragrance allergens in children's cosmetics and cosmetic-toys. *Contact Dermatitis* 41: 84-88.

Rietschel, RL. & Fowler Jr., JF. (2008). Pathogenesis of Allergic Contact Hypersensitivity, In: Rietschel, RL. & Fowler Jr., JF., *Fisher's Contact Dermatitis,* 6th ed., BC Decker Inc, Hamilton, pp. 1-10a.

Rietschel, RL. & Fowler Jr., JF. (2008). Allergic Sensitization to Plants, In: Rietschel, RL. & Fowler Jr., JF, *Fisher's Contact Dermatitis,* 6th ed., BC Decker Inc, Hamilton, pp. 405-453b.

Roul, S., Ducombs, G., Léauté-Labrèze, C. & Taïeb, A. (1998). "Lucky Luke" contact dermatitis due to rubber components of diapers. *Contact Dermatitis* 38: 363-364.

Roul, S., Ducombs, G., Léauté-Labrèze, C., Labbe, L. & Taïeb, A. (1996). Footwear contact dermatitis in children. *Contact Dermatitis* 35: 334-336.

Rudzki, E. & Rebandel, P. (1996). Contact dermatitis in children. *Contact Dermatitis* 34: 66-67.

Rystedt, I. (1985). Contact sensitivity in adults with atopic dermatitis in childhood. *Contact Dermatitis* 13: 1-8.

Salam, TN. & Fowler Jr., JF. (2001). Balsam-related systemic contact dermatitis. *J Am Acad Dermatol* 45: 377-381.

Seidenari, S., Manzini, BM. & Motolese, A. (1992). Contact sensitisation in infants: report of 3 cases. *Contact Dermatitis* 27: 319-320.

Seidenari, S., Giusti, F., Pepe, P. & Mantovani, L. (2005). Contact Sensitization in 1094 Children Undergoing Patch Testing over 7-Year Period. *Pediatr Dermatol* 22: 1-5.

Schnuch, A. & Uter, W. (2003). Decrease in nickel allergy and regulatory interventions. *Contact Dermatitis* 49: 107-108.

Schnuch, A., Uter, W. & Reich, K. (2006). Allergic contact dermatitis and atopic eczema, In: Ring, J., Przybilla, B., Ruzicka, T. (Eds.), *Handbook of Atopic Eczema,* 2nd ed., Springer-Verlag, Berlin, pp. 178-201.

Schnuch, A., Wolter, J., Geier, J. & Uter, W. (2011). Nickel allergy is still frequent in young German females - probably due to insufficient protection from nickel-releasing objects. *Contact Dermatitis* 64: 142-150.

Segurado Rodriguez, MA., Ortiz de Frutos, FJ. & Guerra Tapia, A. (2004). Allergic contact dermatitis. *An Pediatr (Barc)* 60: 599-601.

Senff, H., Exner, M., Görtz, J., Goos, M. (1989). Allergic contact dermatitis from Euxyl K400. *Contact Dermatitis* 20: 381-382, 0105-1873

Shah, M., Lewis, FM. & Gawkrodger, DJ. (1997). Patch testing in children and adolescents: five years' experience and follow-up. *J Am Acad Dermatol* 37: 964-968.

Sosted, H., Hesse, U., Menné, T., Andersen, KE. & Johansen, JD. (2005). Contact dermatitis to hair dyes in an adult Danish population - an interview based study. *Br J Dermatol* 153: 132-135.

Sosted, H., Johansen, JD., Andersen, KE. & Menné, T. (2006). Severe allergic hair dye reactions in 8 children. *Contact Dermatitis* 54: 87-91.

Spann, CT., Tutrone, WD., Weinberg, JM., Scheinfeld, N. & Ross, B. (2003). Topical antibacterial agents for wound care: a primer. *Dermatol Surg* 29: 620-626.

Stables, GI., Forsyth, A. & Lever, RS. (1996). Patch testing in children. *Contact Dermatitis* 34: 341-344.

Thyssen, JP., Johansen, JD., Menné, T., Nielsen, NH. & Linneberg, A. (2009). Nickel allergy in Danish women before and after nickel regulation. *N Engl J Med* 360: 2259-2260.

Thyssen, JP., Uter, W., McFadden, J., Menné, T., Spiewak, R., Vigan, M., Gimenez-Arnau, A. & Lidén, C. (2011). The EU Nickel Directive revisited - future steps towards better protection against nickel allergy. *Contact Dermatitis* 64: 121-125.

Tomar, J., Jain, VK., Aggarwal, K., Dayal, S. & Gupta, S. (2005). Contact allergies to cosmetics: testing with 52 cosmetic ingredients and personal products. *J Dermatol* 32: 951-955.

Tosti, A., Voudouris, S. & Pazzaglia, M. (2003). Contact sensitization to 5-chloro-2-methyl-4-isothiazolin-3-one and 2-methyl-4-isothiazolin-3-one in children. *Contact Dermatitis* 49: 215.

Uhr, JW., Dancis, J. & Neumann, CG. (1960). Delayed-type hypersensitivity in premature neonatal humans. *Nature* 187: 1130-1131.

Uter, W., Ludwig, A., Balda, B-R., Schnuch, A., Pfahlberg, A., Schäfer, T., Wichmann, H-E. & Ring, J. (2004). The prevalence of contact allergy differed between population-based and clinic-based data. *J Clin Epidemiol* 57: 627-632.

Uter, W., Ramsch, C., Aberer, W., Ayala, F., Balato, A., Beliauskiene, A., Fortina, AB., Bircher, A., Brasch, J., Chowdhury, MM., Coenraads, PJ., Schuttelaar, ML., Cooper, S., Corradin, MT., Elsner, P., English, JS., Fartasch, M., Mahler, V., Frosch, PJ., Fuchs, T., Gawkrodger, DJ., Gimènez-Arnau, AM., Green, CM., Horne, HL., Jolanki, R., King, CM., Krêcisz, B., Kiec-Swierczynska, M., Ormerod, AD., Orton,DI., Peserico, A., Rantanen, T., Rustemeyer, T., Sansom, JE., Simon, D., Statham, BN., Wilkinson, M. & Schnuch, A. (2009). The European baseline series in 10 European Countries 2005/2006 - results of the European Surveillance System on Contact Allergies (ESSCA). *Contact Dermatitis* 61: 31-38.

Van Ginkel, CJW. & Rutdervoort, GJ. (1995). Increasing incidence of contact allergy to the new preservative 1,2-dibromo-2,4-dicyanobutane (methyldibromoglutaronitrile). *Br J Dermatol* 132: 918-920.

Vozmediano, F. & Hita, A. (2005). Allergic contact dermatitis in children. *J Eur Acad Dermatol Vevereol* 19: 42-46.

Wahlberg, JE. & Lindgerg, M. (2006). Patch testing, In: Frosch PJ., Menné T. & Lepoittevin JP. (Eds.), *Contact Dermatitis*, 4th ed., Springer-Verlag, Berlin, pp. 366-390.

Wantke, F., Hemmer, W., Jarisch, R. & Götz, M. (1996). Patch test reactions in children, adults and the elderly. A comparative study in patients with suspected allergic contact dermatitis. *Contact Dermatitis* 34: 316-319.

Weston, WL. & Weston, JA. (1984). Allergic contact dermatitis in children. *Am J Dis Child* 138: 932-936.

Weston,WL., Weston, JA., Kinoshita, J., Kloepfer, S., Carreon, L.,Toth, S., Bullard, D., Harper, K. & Martinez, S. (1986). Prevalence of epicutaneous tests among infants, children and adolescents. *Pediatrics* 78: 1070-1074.

White, IR. (2000). Allergic contact dermatitis, In: Harper, J., Oranje, A. & Prose, N. (Eds.), *Textbook of pediatric dermatology*, Vol. 1, Blackwell Science, Oxford, pp. 287-294.

Wöhrl, S., Hemmer, W., Focke, M., Götz, M. & Jarisch, R. (2003). Patch testing in Children, Adults, and the Elderly: Influence of Age and Sex on Sensitization Patterns. *Pediatr Dermatol* 20(2): 119-123.

Worm, A., Aberer,W., Agathos, M., Becker, D., Brasch, J., Fuchs, T., Hillen, U., Höger, P., Mahler, V., Schnuch, A. & Szliska, C. (2007). Patch testing in children - recommendations of the German Contact Dermatitis Research Group (DKG). *J Dtsch Dermatol Ges* 5: 107-109.

8

Contact Dermatitis in Children

Laurel M. Morton and Katherine Szyfelbein Masterpol
Boston University, Department of Dermatology
USA

1. Introduction

Allergic contact dermatitis is increasingly being recognized as a disease that affects children in addition to adults. Historically, irritant contact dermatitis such as 'diaper dermatitis' was a frequent diagnosis made in children, while allergic contact dermatitis was not considered a significant disease in this age group. Clinicians may have attributed this to children's lack of exposure to allergens or to the belief that pediatric immunity was not vigorous enough to result in sensitization. Some suspect that the infrequent diagnosis of this condition was due to scarce patch testing in this age group. It is true that contact allergy has not been studied as intensely in children as in adults and data from adult studies may not always reflect results in children. By means of many reports and epidemiological studies in the literature, it has become clear that allergic contact dermatitis is a significant diagnosis to consider in young children, and even infants, with eczematous disease.

This chapter was written as a review of the current literature. Background regarding allergic contact dermatitis will be provided with a discussion of its prevalence in children. The most common allergens that affect children will be reviewed, and important pearls regarding patch testing will be discussed.

2. Epidemiology

Recent studies suggest that allergic contact dermatitis remains more common in adults than in children (Kwangsukstith & Maibach, 1995) affecting approximately 10% of the adult population (Marks, 1997) and accounting for just over 4% of all dermatologic consultations (Mendenhall et al., 1973). Though the condition is increasingly being recognized in the pediatric population, most epidemiologic studies have been completed retrospectively and investigate the occurrence of positive patch tests in symptomatic patients only. Generally, standard series are used. For example, the European Standard Series is commonly utilized in European studies. Yet, some variation in tested allergens exists and studies often evaluate specific pediatric populations, making it difficult to compare studies. The exact rates of incidence and prevalence remain less clear, potentially due to only recent interest in studying this condition in children. Furthermore, only a minority of studies report on the relevance of positive patch test results.

2.1 Prevalence in infants and young children

A common explanation for low rates of allergic contact dermatitis in children was their lack of a robust immune system. Early studies seemed to support this theory. For instance, Straus found negative patch test results after evaluating 119 infants with poison ivy dermatitis (Straus, 1931). However, in 1960, Uhr and colleagues were able to demonstrate allergic responses to dinitrofluorobenzene in a small series of infants. Of note, premature infants were less likely to have positive reactions compared to infants aged 2-12 months (Uhr et al., 1960). Uhr's study supported that infants could indeed be sensitized, but the younger the infant, the weaker the response. After his work, it would be another twenty years before contact allergy was investigated in children on a broader scale.

The literature now provides numerous studies describing the presence of allergic contact sensitization in very young children. In 1995, Motolese and colleagues reported that up to 60% of symptomatic infants aged 3-24 months elicit positive patch tests (Motolese et al., 1995). Three years later, Manzini and colleagues patch tested a total of 670 children aged 6 months - 12 years old, with suspected disease, and detected positive results in 42% of patients. Furthermore, at least two studies have shown that the highest rate of sensitization occurs in children less than 3 years old (Manzini et al., 1998; Roul et al., 1999). Interestingly, many children (77%) in one such study had concurrent atopic dermatitis, which introduces a much contended issue regarding the relationship between atopic dermatitis and contact dermatitis and whether atopic skin predisposes children to contact allergy (Manzini et al., 1997). In 2003, Wohrl tested 2770 children and adults with suspected disease, finding positive patch tests in 49% of study participants. The highest rate of sensitization was found in children less than 10 years old at a rate of 62% (Wohrl et al., 2003).

There are also many reports that describe the occurrence of allergic contact dermatitis in very young patients, even as young as 1 month of age (Fisher, 1994; Seidenari et al., 1992). This may be related to the fact that infants and children are increasingly exposed to more antigens. This is illustrated by the report of a 5-month-old infant with contact allergy to colophony found in electrocardiogram electrodes used to monitor for sudden infant death syndrome (Oestmann et al., 2007). Or, consider the series of three young children, aged 9 months to 2 years, who developed a diaper dermatitis as a result of disposable diaper dye (Alberta et al., 2005). Such new exposures may, in part, explain the increase in diagnosis of pediatric allergic contact dermatitis.

2.2 Prevalence in symptomatic versus asymptomatic populations

Studies of various sizes attempt to assess the prevalence of pediatric allergic contact dermatitis. However, because of their retrospective nature, most of these studies are limited in that they evaluate symptomatic patients only (Table 1). In the majority of studies, subjects were either suspected of having allergic contact dermatitis or suffered from additional dermatoses including atopic dermatitis and psoriasis. Prevalence in these groups of patients ranges from 14.5% to 83% (Balato et al., 1989; Zug et al., 2008). Though most often, the prevalence is within the range of 40-60%. The most common allergens detected in this setting are nickel, fragrances, cobalt, thimerosal and neomycin. Unfortunately, many of these studies do not indicate the percentage of positive tests that were considered clinically relevant, and this value may be as high as 92% (Rademaker et al., 1989). The responsibility remains with the clinician to determine whether a dermatitis is likely attributable to a contact allergen in the setting of positive test results.

Study	No.	Age	Positive Patch Test	Relevance	Most Frequent Allergens
Brasch & Geier (1997)	416	6-15 yo	40.9%	Not addressed	Nickel sulfate (15.9%) Thimerosal (11.3%) Benzoyl Peroxide (8.9%) Fragrance Mix (8.2%) Cobalt sulfate (7.5%)
Manzini et al. (1998)	670	6mo–12 yo	42%	Not addressed	Thimerosal (23%) Nickel (7.76%) Kathon CG (5.67%) Fragrance Mix (5.52%) Neomycin sulfate (3.58%)
Roul et al. (1999)	337	1-15 yo	66%	Nickel not relevant, Fragrance & Rubber Chemicals relevant	Nickel (23.7%) Fragrance (9.8%) Wool wax alcohols (8.6%) Potassium dichromate (8%) Balsam of peru (4.7%)
Heine et al. (2004)	285 217	6-12 yo 13-18 yo	52.6% 49.7%	Not addressed	Thimerosal (18.2%, 14.3%) Benzoyl Peroxide (16.5%, 8.0%) Phenylmercuric Acetate (13.1%, 7.1%) Gentamicin sulfate (12.5%, 2.9%) Nickel (10.3%, 16.7%)
Seidenari et al. (2005)	1094	7 mo-12 yo	52.1%	Not addressed	Neomycin 20% gel (13.2%) Nickel 5% (10.9%) Wool Alcohols (10.1%) Thimerosal (10.1%) Ammoniated Mercury (8.9%)
Clayton et al. (2006)	500	<16 yo	27%	61%	Nickel (33%) Fragrance Mix (18%) Cobalt (11%) Para-phenylenediamine (8%) Balsam of peru (8%)
Goon et al. (2006)	2340	< 21 yo	45.4%	27 – 83% depending on age and allergen	Nickel (40%) Thimerosal (15%) Colophony (9%) Lanolin (8%) Cobalt (8%)
Zug et al. (2008)	391	0-18 yo	51.2%	Not addressed	Nickel (28.3%) Cobalt Chloride (17.9%) Thimerosal (15.3%) Neomycin (8.0%) Gold Sodium Thiosulfate (7.7%)

Milingou et al. (2010)	232 (1980-93)	< 16 yo	47.8%	Not addressed	Nickel (16.3%) Cobalt Chloride (8.6%) Fragrance Mix (7.3%) Potassium Dichromate (4.3%) Thimerosal (1.7%)
	255 (1994-07)		60%		Nickel (21.56%) Thimerosal (18.03%) Cobalt Chloride (12.9%) Potassium Dichromate (9.4%) Fragrance Mix (4.7%)

Table 1. Prevalence of Allergic Contact Dermatitis in Selected (Symptomatic) Populations (Studies with > 250 patients)

Fewer studies have been completed that investigate the prevalence of allergic contact dermatitis in the general, asymptomatic population (Table 2). One study reported positive

Study	**No.**	**Age**	**Positive Patch Test**	**Most Frequent Allergens**
Weston et al. (1986)	314	<18 yo	20%	Neomycin (8.1%) Nickel (7.6%) Dichromate (7.6%) Thimerosal (3.5%) Balsam of peru (1.5%) Formaldehyde (1.5%)
Barros et al. (1991)	562	Schoolchildren	13.3%	Neomycin Thimerosal PTBPF resin Fragrance Mix
Dotterud & Falk (1995)	424	7-12 yo	23.3%	Nickel (14.9%) Cobalt (5.7%) Kathon CG (5.2%) Lanolin (1.7%) Neomycin (1.4%)
Bruckner et al. (2000)	85	6 mo–5 yo	24.5%	Nickel (12.9%) Thimerosal (9.4%) Kathon CG (2.4%) Neomycin (1.2%) Cobalt (1.2%) *p-tert*-butylphenol (1.2%)
Mortz et al. (2002)	1146	13 yo	15.2%	Nickel (8.6%) Fragrance Mix (1.8%) Colophony (1%) Cobalt Chloride (1%) Thimerosal (1%)

Table 2. Prevalence of Allergic Contact Dermatitis in Unselected (Asymptomatic) Populations

patch test results in 13.3% of 562 schoolchildren. Using this data, investigators suggested that allergic contact dermatitis may be more common than previously suspected (Barros et al., 1991). Weston showed that of 314 healthy children, 20% had at least one positive patch test (Weston et al., 1986). Finally, Bruckner has reported the highest overall prevalence at 24.5% when evaluating 85 healthy patients who presented for routine well-child care visits. In this study, subjects were 6 months to 5 years old, further supporting that young children are not uncommonly sensitized (Bruckner et al., 2000). The most common allergens detected in unselected populations are nickel, thimerosal, neomycin, cobalt, fragrances and Kathon CG (Table 2).

2.3 Prevalence in females versus males

Studies are not consistent with regard to prevalence of pediatric allergic contact dermatitis varying between the sexes. Many suggest that there is no difference (Barros et al., 1991; Bruckner et al., 2000; Weston et al., 1986). Other researchers report that the disease is more prevalent in females (Clayton et al., 2006). Mortz and colleagues reported positive patch tests in 19.4% of unaffected females and 10.35% of unaffected males (Mortz et al., 2002). Giordano-Labadie et al. remark that males and females have a similar overall prevalence of allergic contact dermatitis but that females more commonly show sensitization to nickel in comparison to males (Giordano-Labadie et al., 1999). This sentiment is echoed in other studies, and Beattie reports that up to 82% of positive patch tests to nickel in symptomatic patients occur in females (Beattie et al., 2007; Brasch & Geier, 1997). One reason for this difference between the sexes is likely allergen exposure. Jewelry that contains nickel is more commonly worn by female rather than male children (Modjtahedi et al., 2004). In fact, Jensen and colleagues demonstrated that young Danish girls who had their ears pierced prior to a Danish law that regulated nickel exposure were 3.3 times more likely to display sensitization to nickel compared to females without pierced ears. After regulation, patients were only 1.2 times more likely to be sensitized to nickel if their ears were pierced (Jensen et al., 2002).

2.4 Prevalence as related to culture

When evaluating a patient with suspected allergic contact dermatitis, it is important to consider cultural context. Allergen exposure and age of exposure may vary depending on cultural practices. For example, in a study of 70 symptomatic Indian children, the second-most common allergen was potassium dichromate. Investigators attributed this high prevalence to the frequent use of leather footwear without socks. Another cited cause is the trend towards urbanization in India, which has resulted in exposure to potassium dichromate found in cement and metals. The same article suggests that children may be sensitized to nickel early on due to jewelry that is worn at a young age for religious reasons (Sarma & Ghosh, 2010).

Obtaining the appropriate level of suspicion for an allergic contact dermatitis does not depend on a clinician's complete understanding of a patient's lifestyle or culture, but rather, the clinician's ability to ask the proper questions. Social factors such as job-related exposures are still relevant in the pediatric adolescent population. In one German study, higher rates of sensitization were discovered in adolescents aged 13-18 who worked as hair dressers or in the healthcare field (Heine et al., 2004). Another consideration is the child's hobbies and extracurricular activities. Consider the case of an 11-year-old female cellist with a three year history of an eruption on the right first, second and third digits. She patch tested positive to para-phenylenediamine, which the manufacturer of her bow verified was present in the bow stain (O'Hagan and Bingham, 2001).

2.5 Atopic dermatitis

The association between atopic dermatitis and allergic contact dermatitis remains somewhat unclear. Several older studies that specifically investigated the prevalence of positive patch testing in children with atopic dermatitis suggested that contact allergy is less common in this population (Angelini & Meneghini, 1977). Jones et al. investigated sensitivity to Rhus in atopic and non-atopic patients. Patch tests to Rhus were positive in 61% of healthy patients and only 15% of those with atopic dermatitis (Jones et al., 1973). This correlation may be explained, as contact allergy is a Th1 response and atopic dermatitis patients have a decreased Th1 response (Mortz & Anderson, 1999). Alternatively, some studies suggest that allergic contact dermatitis is more frequent in atopic patients. Epstein and colleagues evaluated the frequency of positive patch tests in patients with atopic dermatitis versus those with psoriasis. Twenty-eight percent of those with atopic dermatitis had positive reactions versus 9% of those with psoriasis (Epstein & Mohajerin, 1964). Another study showed that patch tests were more frequently positive in those with atopic dermatitis versus controls without atopic dermatitis but with other allergic disease including allergic conjunctivitis and asthma (Lammintausta et al., 1992). Dotterud and Falk reported positive tests were significantly more common in schoolchildren with atopic dermatitis, 28.8%, versus 17.9% in controls (Dotterud & Falk, 1995). One explanation for increased risk in atopic patients is their defective skin barrier, which allows for increased exposure to antigens. Also, atopic patients may become sensitized to more allergens given their frequent use of topical agents including emollients, which often contain fragrances and preservatives (Mortz and Anderson, 1999). It should also be considered that atopic skin is readily irritated, which may lead to false positive patch testing results, especially in the case of metals (Dotterud & Falk, 1994). The latter concept is important as some recent studies did not detect a difference in the prevalence of positive patch testing between children with and without atopic dermatitis (Balato et al., 1989; Motolese et al., 1995).

3. Common causes of contact dermatitis in children

3.1 Irritant dermatitis

There are two categories of contact dermatitis that affect the pediatric population: irritant and allergic contact dermatitis. Irritant dermatoses have been diagnosed in children for many years, particularly diaper dermatitis.

3.1.1 Diaper dermatitis

The term 'diaper dermatitis' refers to a multifactorial eruption in the region of the diaper and should not be confused with other diseases that are aggravated by diapers or occur in the same distribution (Scheinfeld, 2005). Factors contributing to primary diaper dermatitis include increased skin moisture and wetness, which create a warm and humid environment that makes infant skin more susceptible to breakdown and more permeable to chemicals and enzymes. An elevated pH results when bacterial ureases split urea in the urine to release ammonia, and this predisposes infant skin to dermatitis. Friction may also play a role, though this is likely a predisposing or exacerbating rather than dominant factor. Fecal enzymes including proteases and lipases have direct irritant action on the skin and their effects are increased by an alkaline environment. Finally, microorganisms, particularly candida, but also staphylococcus, peptostreptococcus, bacteroides, herpes virus, and dermatophytes can worsen irritant diaper dermatitis (Prasad et al., 2003; Wolf et al., 2000).

Other causes of dermatitis in the diaper region include seborrheic dermatitis, psoriasis, atopic dermatitis, congenital syphilis, acrodermatitis enteropathica (zinc deficiency), scabies, child abuse and miliaria. Finally, dermatitis of the diaper area may also be allergic contact dermatitis. Allergens to consider in this setting include sorbitansesquioleate, fragrances (mix I and balsam of peru), disperse dye, cyclohexlthiopthalimide, mercaptobenzothiazole, iodopropylcarbamate, bronopol and *p-tertiary*-butyl-phenol-formaldehyde (Smith & Jacob, 2009).

Prevention and management of irritant diaper dermatitis revolves around keeping the occluded skin dry and limiting the amount of time that the skin is exposed to urine and feces. Removing diapers is one of the oldest and most effective measures in preventing and treating this condition. Frequent diaper changes are most helpful if done immediately after urination and bowel movements (every hour in neonates and every 3-4 hours in infants). Some experts recommend washing the area with mild soap, while others suggest that rinsing the area in lukewarm water is sufficient. New technology has allowed diapers to be much more absorbent and effective in keeping skin dry and with a normal pH. In terms of topical treatments, low potency steroids can be effective for inflamed skin. However, even if these are applied for a short time to acute disease, a waterproof emollient should be placed over them as a barrier to protect the skin. Ideally, emollients should be reapplied after every diaper change. Emollients effective in this setting are usually made of a large quantity of fine powder, such as zinc oxide, suspended in a greasy vehicle. For those eruptions which are superinfected with candida, topical antifungals may also be required (Wolf et al., 2000).

3.1.2 Perianal dermatitis

An entity that is distinct from diaper dermatitis is perianal dermatitis. Fecal components including fecal lipase and bile acids can cause degradation of the skin barrier perianally, leading to an erythematous irritant dermatitis limited to perianal skin (Ruselet-van Embden et al., 2004). There are several less common diagnoses that are thought to be related to irritant perianal dermatitis and some believe that these exist on a spectrum of one disease. These entities include granuloma gluteale infantum, pseudoverrucous papules and Jacquet's erosive dermatitis.

Granuloma gluteale infantum is thought to be multifactorial and related to occlusion, powder, topical halogenated steroids, *Candida* infection, urine and feces. It classically appears as oval, red-purple granulomatous nodules at sites of occlusion (Robson et al., 2006). This condition will improve with removal of inciting agents (Al-Faraidy & Al-Natour, 2010). Pseudoverrucous papules and nodules is a less common condition and was first reported in association with urostomy sites but may also be seen in children in a perianal distribution. Lesions are shiny, smooth, red, moist, flat-topped and round and may be mistaken for condyloma (Robson et al., 2006). Finally, Jacquet's erosive diaper dermatitis describes perianal papules that are well-demarcated, sometimes umbilicated and red-purple in color (2-5mm diameter). They evolve into slow-healing erosions and ulcers (Paradisi et al., 2009) and may have elevated borders (Robson et al., 2006). This usually occurs in infants older than six months. Treatment of this entity can be difficult, but therapeutic options include topical treatment with antibiotics, miconazole, zinc oxide and non-steroidal ant-inflammatory drugs (Paradisi et al., 2009).

3.1.3 Lip-licker's dermatitis

Another relatively common form of irritant dermatitis in children is lip-licker's dermatitis. This presents as erythematous, scaly, thin plaques in a perioral distribution. Characteristically, the vermillion border is involved. It is caused by habitual licking of the lips and skin around the mouth and the irritant in this case is saliva. Atopy, wind and cold weather are predisposing factors. It is managed well with behavioral modification and topical emollients (i.e. petrolatum) acting as barriers from saliva. This entity should be differentiated from perioral dermatitis, which is an eruption of pink scaly papules that generally spares the skin involving the vermillion (Leung & Robson, 2005).

3.2 Allergic contact dermatitis

As mentioned previously, the diagnosis of allergic dermatitis is more frequently being made in children. Tables 1 and 2 list the most common allergens detected in a series of investigations. A recent review evaluates 49 studies, most of which included symptomatic patients, finding the five most common allergens to be nickel sulfate, ammonium persulfate, gold sodium thiosulfate, thimerosal and toluene-2,5-diamine (Bonitsis et al., 2011). Table 3 provides prevalence rates of common allergens.

Allergen	**Prevalence**
Nickel	**5-40%** (Goon et al., 2006; Seidenari et al., 2005)
Mercury	**6.4-25.3%** (Romaguera & Vilaplana, 1998; Wohrl et al., 2003)
Thimerosal	**8.5-23%** (Manzini et al., 1998; Romaguera & Vilaplana, 1998)
Potassium dichromate	**8-21%** (Roul et al., 1999; Wilkowska et al., 1996)
Fragrance	**4.3-19%** (Rademaker & Forsyth, 1989; Romaguera & Vilaplana, 1998)
Cobalt	**3.6-17.9%** (Shah et al., 1997; Zug et al., 2008)
Wool alcohols	**3.58-10.1%** (Manzini et al., 1998; Seidenari et al., 2005)
Rubber chemicals (including carba mix & thiuram)	**4-10%** (Beattie et al., 2007; Fernandez Vozmediano & Armario Hita, 2005)
Balsam of peru	**2.6-8%** (Clayton et al., 2006; Giordano-Labadie et al., 1999)

Table 3. Prevalence of Common Allergens in Selected Populations

3.2.1 Metals

Nickel

Nickel is the most widespread allergen in the general population (Heim & McKean, 2009; Johnke et al., 2004) and is most often identified as the leading allergen in children (Tables 1 & 2). It accounts for up to 14.9% of positive patch tests (Dotterud and Falk, 1995) in asymptomatic children and is generally more frequent in females (Beattie et al., 2007; Brasch & Geier, 1997; Giordano-Labadie et al., 1999). Importantly, young infants may also be sensitized to nickel. In a study of 543 infants followed from birth to age 18 months, 8.6% showed a reproducible positive reaction to this metal (Johnke et al., 2004). Ear piercing is often considered the major risk factor for becoming sensitized to nickel (Smith-Sivertsen et al., 1999). Other sources include everyday items such as jewelry, eyeglass frames, belt buckles, jean snaps, zippers, coins, keys and even cell phones (Hsu et al., 2010). Another potential cause for sensitization is orthodontic devices (Temesvari & Racz, 1988; Veien et al., 1994). In this setting, the allergic contact dermatitis can present as cheilitis, perioral eczema and stomatitis. Other metals are also implicated in this setting including potassium dichromate (Veien et al., 1994). Typical locations for nickel dermatitis include the face, earlobes, wrist, neck and periumbilical skin with the last site being most common (Hsu et al., 2010).

While a localized contact dermatitis is most expected with nickel, id reactions may not be uncommon. Id reaction refers to involvement of skin lacking direct contact with the allergen, resulting from auto-sensitization from circulating immune cells. Such eruptions, sometimes confused with atopic dermatitis, present as pruritic papules distributed on the upper arms, thighs, knees and elbows. They tend to be more persistent than localized contact dermatitis, lasting up to months after localized plaques have cleared (Hsu et al., 2010). Silverberg and colleagues examined 30 pediatric patients with personal history of umbilical or wrist dermatitis or a family history of nickel allergic contact dermatitis. All patients developed a positive patch test to nickel and 50% of patients were reported to develop id reactions (Silverberg et al., 2002). Systemic contact dermatitis has also been reported with nickel. It may present as a generalized dermatitis despite contact with nickel at a limited body site. In some cases, it may result from oral ingestion of nickel, including the small amount that is present in foods and tap water (Hsu et al., 2010).

Cobalt

While a significant percentage of positive patch test results in children are attributed to cobalt, it should be recognized that this metal often co-sensitizes with other metals, particularly nickel and potassium dichromate (Goon & Goh, 2006; Lisi et al., 2003). At times, contamination of cobalt patch tests with nickel may also lead to false positive tests (Lisi et al., 2003). Yet, cobalt itself remains relevant for allergic contact dermatitis. One study attributes 2 of 17 cases of pediatric hand dermatitis to cobalt (Beattie et al., 2007). In 1971, a case was reported of an 11-year-old boy who presented with eczematous lesions at the site of his eyeglass frames, wrists and mouth. His dermatitis was attributed to cobalt in his watch, glasses and the ball point pen that he chewed (Grimm, 1971).

Potassium dichromate

A common source for potassium dichromate exposure in children is its use in tanning leather, particularly in shoes (Sarma and Ghosh, 2010; Weston et al., 1986). In such cases, the distribution of dermatitis is typically located at the dorsal feet and occasionally at the plantar surfaces. Though, if only the plantar surfaces are involved, the diagnosis of juvenile plantar dermatosis should also be considered. Other items that contain potassium dichromate include cement, matches, bleaches, antirust compounds, varnishes, yellow paints, spackling compounds and certain glues (Fisher et al., 2008). While many of these items are encountered more so in occupational exposures, these items could potentially exist in a child's home environment or relate to adolescent hobbies.

Mercury

Sensitization to mercury is relatively common. It is also thought to cross react with thimerosal, a compound that contains mercury. Sources of exposure include shoes in which mercury is used as a preservative, and more classically antiseptic solutions (Fernandez Vozmediano & Armario Hita, 2005). Other items that may contain mercurial agents are eye drops, depigmenting creams, pediculosis preparations, vaccines, broken thermometers, amalgam fillings, contact lens solutions and pesticides (Goossens & Morren, 2004). Another presentation for mercury contact allergy is' baboon syndrome'. This entity was described by Andersen et al. in 1984 and is characterized by a systemic contact dermatitis that involves a pruritic and confluent macular and papular light-red eruption localized to the gluteal cleft and major flexures. It can result from contact with various allergens, but mercury is a classic cause. The most common exposure to mercury has been via inhalation from broken thermometers (Lerch & Bircher, 2004). The use of such thermometers has greatly diminished over the years.

Other metals

Less common metal allergens include aluminum, iron, copper and palladium. The development of pruritic nodules at hyposensitization therapy injection sites has been attributed to aluminum. In one study, 8 of 37 children who underwent this therapy showed a contact allergy to aluminum (Netterlid et al., 2009). Iron is considered a rare cause of allergic contact dermatitis, though one case describing a 7-year-old boy with an iron allergy related to his orthopedic prosthesis has been reported (Hemmer et al., 1996). Copper is also an infrequent allergen, but dental amalgam has been associated with positive copper patch testing thought to be clinically relevant (Wohrl et al., 2003). Allergy to palladium may be attributed to jewelry (Goossens, 2008). In a 1996 study, 7% of 700 adolescents had positive patch tests to palladium. Except for three subjects, they demonstrated positive testing to nickel as well, suggesting co- or cross-sensitization (Kanerva et al., 1996). The importance of palladium alone as a relevant contact allergen is controversial. Similarly, despite a review reporting gold sodium thiosulfate to be a common allergen resulting in positive patch testing, its clinical relevance is debated (Bonitsis et al., 2011). Many who test positive to this allergen can wear gold jewelry without developing a reaction (Andersen & Jensen, 2007).

3.2.2 Pharmaceuticals

Thimerosal

Thimerosal is composed of two allergenic compounds, mercury and thiosalicylic acid, and is among the most common causes for positive patch testing in pediatric studies (Tables 1 & 2). It is used as a preservative in vaccines, antitoxins, ophthalmic preparations, contact lens solutions and eardrops. However, its clinical relevance is often questioned, as most sensitized patients deny a history of dermatitis. High rates of sensitization are likely due to the presence of this compound in mandatory vaccines that were used in the past (Osawa et al., 1991; Schafer et al., 1995). Possibly, thimerosal sensitization is relevant in a subset of children affected by atopic dermatitis. Patrizi and colleagues described a series of five children who developed diffuse atopic dermatitis flares, starting at injection sites, within days of vaccination with thimerosal-containing vaccines. External contamination of the needles is often blamed as a cause for sensitization (Patrizi et al., 1999).

Neomycin

Neomycin is present in many topical preparations including ear and eye drops that are used to treat bacterial infections. In 1979, Leyden and Kligman reported that intermittent use of the agent was not associated with excessive sensitization, as only 1 of 653 subjects less than 12 years old was sensitive to neomycin (Leyden & Kligman, 1979). Since then, however, others have supported its status as a relevant contact allergen (Mortz & Andersen, 1999). In 1986, Weston identified it as the most common allergen causing positive patch test results and attributed this to the prominent use of this agent for bacterial infections and diaper dermatitis (Weston et al., 1986).

Other pharmaceuticals

A number of other pharmaceutical agents and preservatives have been implicated in allergic contact dermatitis, though to a lesser degree than thimerosal and neomycin. These include ethylenediamine, a chemical stabilizer used in Mycolog cream (nystatin and triamcinolone cream) used to treat various skin conditions including diaper dermatitis. It too has been reported as one of the most common causes of positive patch testing in children (Balato et al, 1989). Ethylenediamine can cross react with antihistamines to produce severe systemic reactions. Benzoyl Peroxide is occasionally found among lists of most common allergens (Table 1), but Heine et al. warn that when the adult concentrations of this agent are applied to children during patch testing, false positive reactions can occur due to the agent's irritant potential (Heine et al., 2004). Corticosteroids have been implicated in pediatric allergic contact dermatitis in multiple case reports (Cunha et al., 2003; Luigi et al., 2001). It is recommended that the standard corticosteroid series as well as any agents being used by the child be patch tested when allergic contact dermatitis is suspected in the setting of topical steroid use (Luigi et al., 2001). Less common pharmaceutical allergens have also been reported in children. In 2008, the first case of chlorhexadine allergic contact dermatitis was described in a 4-year-old boy (de Waard-van der Spek & Oranje, 2008). Another case of chlorhexadine contact dermatitis was reported in a 23-month-old with a wound cleaned with this agent. Interestingly, the patient's mother reported that chlorhexadine had been prescribed for umbilical cord care at birth. This case may suggest that sensitization occurred within days to weeks of birth (Le Corre et al., 2010).

3.2.3 Skin care products & fragrances

In present day, cosmetics are being marketed towards children (Kutting et al., 2004). Though industry guidelines exist regarding safe or hypoallergenic compounds, in some instances, these recommendations are not adhered to in made-for-children cosmetics (Rastogi et al.,

1999). Kohl and colleagues patch tested 70 children suspected of having allergic contact dermatitis. In total, 48.6% of them patch tested positive, with cosmetics being the number one cause for sensitization (Kohl et al., 2002). The specific allergens responsible for sensitization in cosmetics are diverse but include fragrances and dyes. Ammonium persulfate and toluene-2,5,diamine are allergens in hair dyes, and interestingly, children often patch test positive to these agents (Bonitsis et al., 2007). Preservatives, including formaldehyde and formaldehyde releasers, are also considered relevant allergens in cosmetics, with Kathon CG being the most common preservative to patch test positive in one study (Conti et al., 1997). Interestingly, not all of children's exposure to cosmetics is direct, but may be related to agents used by caretakers. Fisher reported a 7-year-old girl with an allergy to cinnamic aldehyde who presented with cheilitis and periorbital dermatitis caused by her mother's lipstick (Fisher, 1995).

Symptomatic children frequently exhibit positive patch testing to fragrances, as elucidated by several recent studies (Clayton et al., 2006; Hogeling & Pratt, 2008; Milingou et al., 2010; Zug et al., 2010). A particularly important diagnostic tool is the 'Fragrance Mix' patch test, which contains three cinnamic derivatives, two eugenol derivatives, geraniol, hydroxycitronellal and oak moss absolute extract. Fragrances are nearly ubiquitous, as they are present in many products including cosmetics, toiletries, soaps, laundry detergents, cleansers, rubber, plastic, paper and textiles (Johansen, 2002). Allergic contact dermatitis due to fragrances may present in either a localized or generalized distribution, and facial dermatitis is more common in those with fragrance contact allergy compared to those without. In adolescent patients, axillary exanthem may indicate a fragrance allergy due to use of deodorants (Johansen, 2002).

Balsam of peru is a plant-derived allergen that is present in many topical medications and cosmetics due to its aromatic properties. It has marginal bacteriocidal activity and is used in toothpastes, cough lozenges and dental cements. It is not an uncommon cause of sensitization in infants and children (Fisher et al., 2008) and is found to be one of the most frequent causes of positive patch testing in children (Kuiters et al., 1989; Jacob et al., 2008; Romaguera et al., 1998; Roul et al., 1999). The face is a common site of involvement (Edman, 1985).

Other rising causes of allergic contact dermatitis, which could be avoided in children, are natural remedies. Oftentimes, these agents are presumed safe because they are 'natural' but in fact, several have been linked to dermatitis (Kutting et al., 2004). For example, tea tree oil derived from the Melaleuca alternifolia cheel is considered a treatment for many skin conditions including infections and acne (Allen, 2001; Bedi & Shenefelt, 2002). It contains approximately 100 components which are generally in low enough concentrations so as not to induce allergy (Kutting et al., 2004). However, when photoaged, tea tree oil becomes a stronger sensitizer due to formation of monoterpene breakdown products (Hausen et al., 1999).

Another skin care product particularly pertinent to the field of dermatology is sunscreen. Much data regarding the allergic potential of sunscreens is in adults. However, there are multiple agents which are reported to cause contact allergy in children as well. Though photoallergy is generally uncommon in children, Cook and Freeman described a case of photoallergic contact dermatitis to two sunscreen agents, methoxycinnamate and oxybenzone, in a 6-year-old (Cook & Freeman, 2002). Recently, octocrylene, a solar filter from the cinnamate family, has been used as a sunscreen against UVB and near-UVA range. It was initially considered to be non-allergenic (Delplace & Blondeel, 2006). But even this agent has caused positive patch tests in 10 of 11 children tested (Avenel-Audran et al., 2010). Not all sunscreen ingredients that can cause allergy are active ingredients. Chu and Sun reported a case of contact allergy to triethanolamine, an emulsifier in sunscreens, in an 8-year-old girl (Chu & Sun, 2001).

A somewhat controversial allergen in adults and children is lanolin, containing wool alcohols. It is found in many skin care products such as Aquaphor Healing Ointment ® (AHO), an emollient commonly used in atopic children. Though previously thought to be a pertinent allergen, in 1998, Kligman wrote that lanolin was "at most a weak contact allergen" and that many case reports represented false positives (Kligman, 1998). However, a few large scale epidemiologic studies list wool alcohols as one of the most common allergens in children (Tables 1 and 2). Epidemiologic data in adults suggests that over time, positive patch testing to lanolin is in fact decreasing (Warshaw et al., 2009). However, in 2010, Matiz and Jacob reported that at least two children who reported burning or irritation to AHO and tested negative to commercially prepared lanolin (one to the T.R.U.E. test and one to Allergeaze) also tested positive to lanolin 30% in petrolatum (Beiersdorf) and their own AHO product (Matiz & Jacob, 2010). These conflicting opinions may not be cause to stop recommending agents that contain lanolin, but rather, a reason for suspicion of allergy if parents report a reaction or if a patient's dermatitis is not improving.

3.2.4 Rubber chemicals

Natural rubber (latex) itself is most often associated with a type I hypersensitivity reaction, which is characterized by urticaria and, in severe cases, anaphylaxis. However, many rubber additives are responsible for type IV hypersensitivity in the form of allergic contact dermatitis. These include accelerators such as thiurams, carbamates, thioureas and mercaptobenzothiazoles (MBTs) and antioxidants such as para-phenylenediamine (PPD) derivatives, which retard environmental degradation (Fisher et al., 2008.) These additives can result in a variety of clinical presentations. The face may be affected after contact with balloons. Eruptions at the waistline have occurred in response to elastic underwear and rubber sponges. Balls and gloves may cause chronic hand eczema (Goossens & Morren, 2004).There is also at least one case report of co-existent type I and type IV sensitivity to rubber latex in a 6-year-old dental patient (Placucci et al., 1996)).

In Beattie et al's study, it was reported that thiuram mix and PPD were each responsible for one case of hand dermatitis (from a total of 17 cases). In the same study, of five cases of foot dermatitis with relevant positive patch tests, two were attributed to mercapto mix and MBT and one to PPD. Such dermatoses are attributed to the presence of these agents in rubber shoe components. Shoe dermatitis that is attributed to allergic contact typically presents as a pruritic papular exanthem on the dorsum of the toes, sparing the webspaces (Sharma &Asati, 2010).

A new pattern for allergic contact dermatitis has been attributed to anti-leak diapers, which feature elastic bands at the thighs that are quite tight. These diapers cause a characteristic distribution of dermatitis at the outer buttocks and hips in toddlers, which resembles a gunbelt holster. The term 'Lucky Luke' is used to describe this entity that has been attributed to MBT, BPF (Roul et al., 1998) and recently cyclohexylthiophathalimide, which is used as a vulcanization retarder in rubber (Belhadjali et al., 2001).

3.2.5 Plants

Plants, particularly those of the Rhus family, are often thought of in the context of allergic contact dermatitis, though they are infrequently within the top five allergens detected in children (Table 1). Up to 85% of the population is sensitized to plants within the Toxicodendron genus, which includes poison ivy, and most patients are sensitized between ages 8 and 14 years old (Koo et al., 2010). Plant allergy can often be identified by history and distribution generally at exposed sites. *Rhus verniiciflua* (Japanese lacquer tree) has been reported in children to cause severe allergic contact dermatitis, which can be mistaken for cellulitis. Many reported patients required systemic steroids due to severity of rash (Gach et al., 2006; Rademaker & Duffill, 1995).

Compositae (Asteraceae) is the second largest plant family and is a well-recognized cause for contact allergy in gardeners, florists and farmers due to the sesquiterpene lactone component. For some time, it was rarely considered a clinically relevant allergen in children. However, there are several cases described in the literature. Flohr and colleagues described hand dermatitis in three children aged 3-8 years old, each of whom had frequent exposure to plants and tested positive to Compositae (Flohr et al., 2008). Paulsen et al. suggest that this particular allergy may be more common in atopic patients (Paulsen et al., 2008.) and Belloni Fortina et al. propose it should be added to the pediatric screening series when investigating airborne dermatitis in atopic children. They made this recommendation after finding 12 of 641 children sensitized to this antigen (Belloni Fortina et al., 2005).

3.2.6 Henna tattoos with para-phenylenediamine (PPD)

Henna (*Lawsoniainermis*) is a plant from the Lythraceae family. Henna dye is a dark green powder made from the leaves of this plant and used for hair dyeing and for temporary body tattooing. PPD is added to henna dye in order to make the color darker and speed the dyeing process (Jovanovic & Slavkovi-Jovanovic, 2009). This tattooing practice is becoming more popular in the pediatric population. PPD is a potent sensitizer and the literature is peppered with case reports regarding sensitization to PPD after henna tattooing in children (Jovanovic & Slavkovi-Jovanovic, 2009; Sidwell et al., 2008). As this exposure is becoming more prevalent in the pediatric population, some are calling for increased regulations (Sidwell et al., 2008).

4. Utility of patch testing

With increasing recognition of allergic contact dermatitis in the pediatric population, patch testing is becoming more important in this age group. Relative to the total number of studies investigating the prevalence of positive patch testing, those which address clinical relevance of results are fewer. However, a number of epidemiologic studies reflect upon the significance of positive tests, supporting the use of this diagnostic modality in pediatrics. In 1989, Kuiter reported that over 23% of positive tests were clinically relevant, while

Rademaker purported that the value was as high at 92% (Kuiters et al., 1989; Rademaker et al., 1989). A review of studies that report on relevance suggests that the value is probably around 60% (Table 1). Many authors specifically endorse the use of patch testing in children (Jacob et al., 2008; Worm et al., 2007). In the past, it was recommended that the concentration of patch tests be reduced in children (Fisher, 1975; Hjorth, 1981). For example, Fisher recommended using half the recommended concentration (Fisher, 1975). This was due the concern that children are at higher risk of developing irritant reactions and thus, false positive tests (Mortz & Andersen, 1999). However, recent studies suggest that the incidence of irritant reactions is low. Brasch and Geier reported a 9% incidence of irritant reactions (Brasch & Geier, 1997). Most experts recommend the use of the same allergen concentration in children as in adults (Brasch & Geier, 1997; Mortz & Andersen, 1999; Roul et al., 1997; Worm, 2006).

Multiple groups recommend abbreviated series in children, in part due to smaller body surface area of normal skin on which to perform the testing. The German Contact Dermatitis Research Group suggests that in children aged 6-12 years old, the following allergens should be tested: nickel sulfate, thiuram mix, colophony, mercaptobenzothiazole, fragrance mix I, fragrance mix II, mercapto mix, bufexamac, dibromodicyanobutane, chlor-methylisothiazolinone, neomycin and Compositae mix. Potassium dichromate, wool alcohols, disperse blue mix, para-phenylenediamine and *p-tert.*-butylphenol-formaldehyde resin may be added if clinically indicated (Worm et al., 2007). Brasch and Geier advocate for a shorter series that includes nickel, cobalt, dichromate, thimerosal, fragrance allergens, wool wax alcohols and Kathon CG. Their analysis was conducted in Germany, and they suggest that since different geographic locations may show varying rates of sensitization to allergens, local experience should be considered when choosing patch testing series for children (Brasch & Geier, 1997). Finally, Seidenari et al. advise clinicians to use patch testing in children but warn that due to frequent changes in relevant allergen exposures, periodic evaluations of the appropriate testing trays should be done for the pediatric population (Seidenari et al., 2005).

Of note, it should be mentioned that while patch testing often yields positive results to relevant allergens, it is unclear that finding a positive allergen is associated with improved clinical outcome. This is generally due to lack of data. Moustafa et al. recently published retrospective data supporting the relevance of positive patch tests in 44% of 110 children. Unfortunately, finding a positive allergen was not associated with improved clinical outcome in this population (Moustafa et al., 2011).

In adults, it has been shown that performing delayed patch test readings often yields more positive results. Matiz and colleagues have recently proposed that this is true in children as well. In 38 children aged 6 -17 years old, patch tests were evaluated after 48 hours, 72-96 hours and again at 7-9 days. 50% of children revealed positive reactions at the 7-9 day mark and 13% of the total number of children revealed new late delayed reactions. 4 of 6 late delayed allergens were considered clinically relevant including quaternium 15, formaldehyde, diazolidinyl urea and *p-tert*-butylphenol formaldehyde resin (Matiz et al., 2011). While this may not be a feasible approach to patch testing in all patients, it is a useful pearl in children for whom a diagnosis of allergic contact dermatitis is highly suspected.

Perioral	Nickel, potassium dichromate, cobalt, amalgam fillings (mercury), flavoring agents (cinnamic aldehyde)
Periorbital	Ophthalmic preparations (mercury, thimerosal)
Face	Topical pharmaceuticals (benzoyl peroxide, sunscreen allergens), fragrances including balsam of peru, nickel
Ears	Otic preparations (thimerosal, neomycin), nickel, cobalt
Neck	Nickel, fragrance
Wrists	Nickel, cobalt, potassium dichromate
Hands	Nickel, cobalt, rubber additives (including thiuram and PPD), plants (Rhus)
Arms	Vaccines (mercury, thimerosal), hyposensitization therapy (aluminum), sunscreen allergens
Feet	Potassium dichromate
Periumbilical	Nickel
Diaper area	Topical pharmaceuticals (neomycin, ethylenediamine), rubber additives
Trunk, Extremities	PPD, clothing dyes, sunscreen allergens, plants

Table 4. Patterns of Localization of Allergic Contact Dermatitis and Their Respective Allergens.

5. Conclusion

As clinicians begin to recognize the diagnosis of allergic contact dermatitis in children, they should also appreciate that the approach to this disease must be different than in adults. The allergens to which children are exposed are often not the same as those that can affect adults. The use of patch testing may be helpful in this age group, but may need to be modified to evaluate for the most clinically relevant allergens. The body of research that is conducted in this area of dermatology continues to grow and it seems likely that our understanding of allergic contact dermatitis in children will continue to advance as will our ability to diagnose and manage this condition. In particular, further epidemiologic studies in asymptomatic patients that focus on the relevance of positive patch test results will be helpful.

6. References

Alberta L, Sweeney SM, Wiss K. Diaper Dye Dermatitis. Pediatrics.2005; 116: e450-2.

Al-Faraidy NA, Al-Natour SH. A forgotten complication of diaper dermatitis: Granuloma gluteale infantum. Journal of Family and Community Medicine. 2010; 17: 107-9.

Allen P. Tea tree oil: the science behind the antimicrobial hype. The Lancet. 2001; 358: 1245.

Andersen KE, Hjorth N, Menne T. The baboon syndrome: systemically-induced allergic contact dermatitis. Contact Dermatitis. 1984; 10: 97-100.

Andersen KE, Jensen CD. Long-lasting patch reactions to gold sodium thiosulfate occur frequently in healthy volunteers. Contact Dermatitis. 2007; 56: 214-7.

Angelini G, Meneghini CL. Contact and bacterial allergy in children with atopic dermatitis. Contact Dermatitis. 1977; 3: 163-7.

Avenel-Audran M, Dutarte H, Goossens A, Jeanmougin M, Comte C, Bernier C, et al. Octocrylene, an emerging photoallergen. Archives of Dermatology. 2010; 146: 753-7.

Ayala F, Balato N, Lembo G, Patruno C, Tosti A, Schena D, et al.A multicenter study of contact sensitization in children .Gruppo Italiano Ricerca Dermatiti da Contatto e Embientali (GIRDCA). Contact Dermatitis. 1992; 26: 307-10.

Balato N, Lembo G, Patruno C, Ayala F. Patch testing in children. Contact Dermatitis. 1989; 20: 305-7.

Barros MA, Baptista A, Correia TM, Azevedo F. Patch Testing in children: a study of 562 schoolchildren. Contact Dermatitis. 1991; 25: 156-9.

Beattie PE, Green C, Lowe G, Lewis-Jones MS. Which children should be patch tested? Clinical and Experimental Dermatology. 2007; 32: 6-11.

Bedi MK, Shenefelt PD. Herbal therapy in dermatology. Archives of Dermatology. 2002; 138: 232-42.

Belhadjali H, Giordano-Labadie F, Rance F, Bazex J. "Lucky Luke" contact dermatitis from diapers: a new allergen? Contact Dermatitis. 2001; 44: 248.

BelloniFortina A, Romano I, Peserico A. Contact sensitization to Compositae mix in children. Journal of the American Academy of Dermatology. 2005; 53: 877-80.

Bonitsis NG, Tatsioni A, Bassioukas K, Ionnidis JPA. Allergens responsible for allergic contact dermatitis among children: a systematic review and meta-analysis. Contact Dermatitis. 2011; 64: 245-57.

Brasch J, Geier J. Patch test results in schoolchildren. Results from the Information Network of Departments of Dermatology (IVDK) and the German Contact Dermatitis Research Group (DKG). Contact Dermatitis. 1997; 37: 286-93.

Bruckner AL, Weston WL, Morelli JG. Does Sensitization to Contact Allergens Begin in Infancy? Pediatrics. 2000; 105: e3.

Bruckner AL, Weston WL. Allergic contact dermatitis in children: a practical approach to management. Skin Therapy Letter. 2002; 7: 3-5.

Carbone A, Siu A, Patel R. Pediatric Atopic Dermatitis: A Review of the Medical Management. The Annals of Pharmacotherapy. 2010; 44: 1448-58.

Chu C, Sun C. Allergic contact dermatitis from triethanolamine in a sunscreen. Contact Dermatitis. 2001; 44: 41-2.

Clayton TH, Wilkinson SM, Rawcliffe C, Pollack B, Clark SM. Allergic contact dermatitis in children: should pattern of dermatitis determine referral? A retrospective study of 500 children tested between 1995 and 2004 in one U.K. center. British Journal of Dermatology. 2006; 154: 114- 7.

Conti A, Motolese A, Manzini BM, Seidenari S. Contact sensitization to preservatives in children. Contact Dermatitis. 1997; 37: 35-6.

Cook N, Freeman S. Photosensitive dermatitis due to sunscreen allergy in a child. Australasian Journal of Dermatology. 2002; 43: 133-5.

Cunha AP, Mota AV, Barros MA, Bonito-Victor A, Resende C. Corticosteroid contact allergy from a nasal spray in a child. Contact Dermatitis. 2003; 48: 277.

Delplace D, Blondeel A. Octocrylene: really non-allergenic? Contact Dermatitis. 2006; 54: 295.

deWaard-van der Spek FB, Oranje AP. Allergic contact dermatitis to chlorhexadine and para-amino compounds in a 4-year-old boy: a very rare observation. Contact Dermatitis. 2008; 58: 239-41.

deWaard-van der Spek FB, Oranje AP. Patch tests in children with suspected allergic contact dermatitis: a prospective study and review of the literature. Dermatology. 2009; 218: 119-225

Dotterud LK, Falk ES. Metal allergy in north Norwegian schoolchildren and its relationship with ear piercing and atopy. Contact Dermatitis. 1994; 31: 303-13

Dotterud LK, Falk ES. Contact allergy in relation to hand eczema and atopic diseases in north Norwegian schoolchildren. Actapaediatrica. 1995; 84: 402-6.

Duarte I, Lazzarini R, Kobata CM. Contact dermatitis in adolescents. American Journal of Contact Dermatitis. 2003; 14: 200-2.

Edman B. Sites of contact dermatitis in relationship to particular allergens. Contact Dermatitis. 1985; 13: 129-35.

Epstein S, Mohajerin AH. Incidence of Contact Sensitivity in Atopic Dermatitis. Archives of Dermatology. 1964; 90: 284-7.

Farage MA, Berardesca E, Maibach H. The possible relevance of sex hormones on irritant and allergic responses: their importance for skin testing. Contact Dermatitis. 2010; 62: 67-74.

Fernandez Vozmediano JM, Armario Hita JC. Allergic contact dermatitis in children. Journal of the European Academy of Dermatology and Venereology. 2005; 19: 42-6.

Fisher AA. Allergic contact dermatitis in early infancy. Cutis. 1994; 54: 300-2.

Fisher AA. Childhood allergic contact dermatitis. Cutis. 1975; 15: 635-42.

Fisher AA. Cosmetic dermatitis in childhood. Cutis. 1995; 55: 15-6.

Flohr C, Ravenscroft J, English J. Compositae allergy in three children with hand dermatitis. Contact Dermatitis. 2008; 59: 370.

Freeman S. Shoe dermatitis. Contact Dermatitis. 1997; 36: 247-51.

Gach JE, Tucker W, Hill VA. Three cases of severe Rhus dermatitis in an English primary school. Journal of the European Academy of Dermatology and Venereology. 2006; 20: 212-3.

Giordano-Labadie F, Rance F, Pellegrin F, Bazex J, Dutau G, Schwarze HP. Prevalence of contact allergy in children with atopic dermatitis: results of a prospective study of 137 cases. Contact Dermatitis. 1999; 40: 192-5.

Goncalo S, Goncalo M, Azenha A, Barros MA, Bastos AS, Brandao FM, et al. Allergic contact dermatitis in children. A multicenter study of the Portuguese Contact Dermatitis Group (GPEDC). Contact Dermatitis. 1993; 26: 112-5.

Goon AT, Goh C. Patch Testing of Singapore Children and Adolescents: Our Experience over 18 Years. Pediatric Dermatology. 2006; 23: 117-20.

Goossens A. The allergens in children. Contact Dermatitis. 2008; 58 Suppl 1: 9-30.

Grimm I. Unusual form of a contact dermatitis due to cobalt in an 11-year-old child. Berufsdermatosen. 1971; 19: 39-42.

Hausen BM, Reichling J, Harkenthal M. Degradation products of monoterpenes are the sensitizing agents in tea tree oil. American Journal of Contact Dermatitis. 1999; 10: 68-77.

Heim KE, McKean BA. Children's clothing fasteners as a potential source of exposure to releasable nickel ions. Contact Dermatitis. 2009; 60: 100-5.

Heine G, Schnuch A, Uter W, Worm M. Frequency of contact allergy in German children and adolescents patch tested between 1995 and 2002: results from the Information Network of Departments of Dermatology and the German Contact Dermatitis Research Group. Contact Dermatitis. 2004; 51: 111-7.

Hemmer W, Focke M, Wantke F, Gotz M, Jarisch R. Contact hypersensitivity to iron. Contact Dermatitis. 1996; 34: 219-20.

Hjorth N. Contact dermatitis in children. Actadermato-venereologica (Stockh). 1981; 95: 36-9.

Hogeling M, Pratt M. Allergic contact dermatitis in children: the Ottawa hospital patch-testing clinic experience, 1996 to 2006. Dermatitis. 2008; 19: 86-89.

Hsu JW, Matiz C, Jacob SE. Nickel Allergy: Localized, Id, and Systemic Manifestations in Children. Pediatric Dermatology. 2011; 28: 276-80.

Jacob SE, Brod B, Crawford GH. Clinically Relevant Patch Test Reactions in Children - A United States Based Study. Pediatric Dermatology. 2008; 25: 520-7.

Jensen CS, Lisby S, Baadsgaard O, Volund A, Menne T. Decrease in nickel sensitization in a Danish schoolgirl population with ears pierced after implementation of nickel-exposure regulation. British Journal of Dermatology. 2002; 146: 636-42.

Johansen JD. Contact allergy to fragrances: clinical and experimental investigations of the fragrance mix and its ingredients. Contact Dermatitis. 2002; 46 Suppl 3: 1-31.

Johnke H, Norberg LA, Vach W, Bindslev-Jensen C, Host A, Andersen KE. Reactivity to patch tests with nickel sulfate and fragrance mix in infants. Contact Dermatitis. 2004; 51: 141-7.

Jones HE, Lewis CW, McMarlin SL. Allergic contact sensitivity in atopic dermatitis. Archives of Dermatology. 1973; 107: 217-22.

Jovanovic DL, Slavkovi-Jovanovic MR. Allergic contact dermatitis from temporary henna tattoo. Journal of Dermatology. 2009; 36: 63-5.

Kalish RS. Recent Developments in the Pathogenesis of Allergic Contact Dermatitis. Archives of Dermatology. 1991; 127: 1558-63.

Kanerva L, Kerosuo H, Kullaa A, Kerosuo E. Allergic patch test reactions to palladium chloride in schoolchildren. Contact Dermatitis. 1996; 34: 39-42.

Kerosuo H, Kullaa A, Kerosuo E, Kanerva L, Hensten-Pettersen A. Nickel allergy in adolescents in relation to orthodontic treatment and piercing of ears. American Journal of Orthodontics and Dentofacial Orthopedics. 1996; 109: 148-54.

Kligman AM. The myth of lanolin allergy. Contact Dermatitis. 1998; 39: 103-7.

Kohl L, Blondeel A, Song M. Allergic contact dermatitis from cosmetics. Retrospective analysis of 819 patch-tested patients. Dermatology. 2002; 204: 334-7.

Koning H, Baert MRM., Oranje AP, Savelkoul HF, Neijeng HJ. Development of immune functions related to allergic mechanisms in young children. Pediatric Research. 1996; 40: 363-75.

Koo B, Leib JA, Garzon MC, Morel KD. Five-year-old Body with a Diffuse Erythematous rash with Black Crusts. Pediatric Dermatology. 2010; 27: 395-6.

Kuiters GR, Smitt JH, Cohen EB, Bos JD. Allergic contact dermatitis in children and young adults. Archives of Dermatology. 1989; 125: 1531-3.

Kutting B, Brehler R, Traupe H. Allergic contact dermatitis in children - strategies of prevention and risk management. European Journal of Dermatology. 2004; 14: 80-5.

Kwangsukstith C, Maibach HI. Effect of age and sex on the induction and elicitation of allergic contact dermatitis. Contact Dermatitis. 1995; 33: 289-98.

Lammintausta K, Kalimo K, Fagerlund VL. Patch test reactions in atopic patients. Contact Dermatitis. 1992; 26: 234-40.

Larsson-Stymne B, Widstrom L. Ear piercing - a cause of nickel allergy in schoolgirls? Contact Dermatitis. 1985; 13: 289-93.

Le Corre Y, Barbarot S, Frot AS, Milpied B. Allergic Contact Dermatitis to Chlorhexidine in a Very Young Child. Pediatric Dermatology. 2010; 27: 485-7.

Lerch M, Bircher AJ. Systemically induced allergic exanthem from mercury. Contact Dermatitis. 2004; 50: 349-53.

Leung AKC, Robson LM. Factitious Dermatitis: Lip Licker's Dermatitis. Consultant 360. 2005; 45: 2.

Lewis VJ, Statham BN, Chowdhury MMU. Allergic contact dermatitis in 191 consecutively patch tested children. Contact Dermatitis. 2004; 51: 155-6.

Leyden JJ, Kligman AM. Contact dermatitis to neomycin sulfate. Journal of the American Medical Association. 1979; 242: 1276-8.

Lisi P, Brunelli L, Stingeni L. Co-sensitivity between cobalt and other transition metals. Contact Dermatitis. 2003; 48: 172-3.

Luigi A, Massimiliano N, Suppa F. Contact sensitivity to budesonide in a child. Contact Dermatitis. 2000; 42: 359.

Manzini BM, Ferdani G, Simonetti V, Donini M, Seidenari S. Contact Sensitization in Children. Pediatric Dermatology. 1998; 15: 12-17.

Marcussen PV. Primary Irritant Patch-Test Reactions in Children. Archives of Dermatology.1963; 87: 378-82.

Marks JG, DeLeo VA. Contact and Occupational Dermatology. 2nd ed. St Louis: Mosby; 1997.

Matiz C, Russell K, Jacob SE. The Importance of Checking for Delayed Reactions in Pediatric Patch Testing. Pediatric Dermatology. 2011; 28: 12-4.

Matiz C, Hsu JW, Paz Castanedo-Tardan M, Jacob SE. Allergic contact dermatitis in children: a review of international studies. GionaleItaliano di dermatologia e venereologia. 2009; 144: 541-56.

Matiz C, Jacob SE. The lanolin paradox revisited. Journal of American Academy of Dermatology. 2010; 64: 197.

Mendenhall RC, Ramsay DL, Girard RA, DeFlorio GP, Weary PE, Lloyd JS. A study of the practice of dermatology in the United States. Initial findings. Archives of Dermatology. 1973; 114: 1456-62

Milingou M, Tagka A, Armenaka M, Kimouri K, Kouismintzis D, Katsarou A. Patch tests in children: a review of 13 years of experience in comparison with previous data. Pediatric Dermatology. 2010; 27: 255-9.

Modjtahedi BS, Modjtahedi SP, Maibach HI. The sex of the individual as a factor in allergic contact dermatitis. Contact Dermatitis. 2004; 50: 53-9.

Mortz CG, Andersen KE. Allergic contact dermatitis in children and adolescents. Contact Dermatitis. 1999; 41: 121-30.

Mortz CG, Lauritsen JM, Bindslev-Jensen C, Andersen KE. Contact Allergy and Allergic Contact Dermatitis in Adolescents: Prevalence Measures and Associations. ActaDermato-Venereologica. 2002; 82: 352-8

Moustafa M, Holden CR, Athavale P, Cork MJ, Messenger AG, Gawkrodger DJ. Patch testing is a useful investigation in children with eczema. Contact Dermatitis. Epub 2011 Apr 19.

Motolese A, Manzini BM, Donini M. Patch testing in infants. American Journal of Contact Dermatitis. 1995; 6: 153-6.

Netterlid E, Hindsen M, Bjork J, Ekovist S, Guner N, Henricson KA, Bruze M. There is an association between contact allergy to aluminum and persistent subcutaneous nodules in children undergoing hyposensitization therapy. Contact Dermatitis. 2009; 60: 41-9

Oestmann E, Phillipp S, Zuberbier T, Worm M. Colophony-induced contact dermatitis due to ECG electrodes in an infant. Contact Dermatitis. 2007; 56: 177-8.

Ogra PL, Welliver RC. Effects of early environment on mucosal immunologic homeostasis, subsequent immune responses and disease outcome. Nestle Nutrition Workshop Series. Paediatricprogramme. 2008; 61: 145-81.

O'Hagan AH, Bingham EA. Cellist's finger dermatitis. Contact Dermatitis. 2001; 45: 319.

Osawa J, Kitamura K, Ikezawa Z, Nakajima H. A probable role for vaccines containing thiomersal in thiomersalhypersensitivity. Contact Dermatitis. 1991; 24: 178-82.

Paradisi A, Capizzi R, Ghitti F, Lanza-Silveri S, Rendeli C, Guerriero C. Jacquet erosive diaper dermatitis: a therapeutic challenge. Clinical and Experimental Dermatology. 2009; 34: e385-6.

Patrizi A, Rizzoli L, Vincenzi C, Trevisi P, Tosti A. Sensitization to thimerosal in atopic children. Contact Dermatitis. 1990; 40: 94-7.

Paulsen E, Otkjjaer A, Andersen KE. Sesquiterpene lactone dermatitis in the young: is atopy a risk factor? Contact Dermatitis. 2008; 59: 1-6.

Pevny I, Brennenstuhl M, Razinskas G. Patch testing in children. (I) Collective test results; skin testability in children. Contact Dermatitis. 1984; 11: 201-6.

Pigatto P, Martelli A, Marsili C, Fiocchi A. Contact Dermatitis in Children. Italian Journal of Pediatrics. 2010; 36: 2.

Placucci F, Vincenzi C, Ghedini G, Piana G, Tosti A. Coexistence of type 1 and type 4 allergy to rubber latex. Contact Dermatitis. 1996; 34: 118.

Prasad HRY, Srivastava P, Verma KK. Diaper dermatitis – An overview. Indian Journal of Pediatrics. 2003; 70: 635-7.

Rademaker M, Duffill MB. Allergic contact dermatitis to Toxicodendron succedaneum (rhus tress): an autumn epidemic. New Zealand Medical Journal. 1995; 108: 121-3.

Rademaker M, Forsyth A. Contact dermatitis in children. Contact Dermatitis. 1989; 20: 104-7.

Rastogi SC, Johansen JD, Menne T, Frosch P, Bruze M, Andersen KE, et al. Contents of fragrance allergens in chidren's cosmetics and cosmetic-toys. Contact Dermatitis. 1999; 41: 84-8.

Rietschel RL, Fowler JF. Fisher's Contact Dermatitis. 6th ed. Ontario: BC Decker, Inc; 2008.

Robson KJ, Maughan JA, Purcell SD, Petersen MJ, Haefner HK, Lowe L. Erosive papulonodular dermatosis associated with topical benzocaine: A report of two cases and evidence that granuloma gluteale, pseudoverrucous papules, and Jacquet's erosive dermatitis are a disease spectrum. Journal of the American Academy of Dermatology. 2006; 55 Suppl 5: S74-80.

Romaguera C, Vilaplana J. Contact dermatitis in children: 6 years experience. Contact Dermatitis. 1998; 39: 277-80

Roul S, Ducombs G, Leaute-Labreze C, Taieb A. 'Lucky Luke' contact dermatitis due to rubber components of diapers. Contact Dermatitis. 1998; 38: 363-4.

Roul S, Ducombs G, Taieb A. Usefulness of the European standard series for patch testing in children. Contact Dermatitis. 1990; 40: 232-5.

Ruseler-van Embden JGH, van Lieshout LMC, Smits SA, van Kessel I, Laman JD. Potato tuber proteins efficiently inhibit human faecal proteolytic activity: implications for treatment of peri-anal dermatitis. European Journal of Clinical Investigation. 2004; 34: 303-11.

Sarma N, Ghosh S. Clinico-allergological pattern of allergic contact dermatitis among 70 Indian children. Indian Journal of Dermatology,Venereology and Leprology. 2010; 76: 38-44.

Schafter T, Enders F, Przybilla B. Sensitization to thimerosal and previous vaccination. Contact Dermatitis. 1995; 32: 114-6.

Scheinfeld N. Diaper dermatitis: a review and brief survey of eruptions of the diaper area. American journal of clinical dermatology. 2005; 6: 273-81.

Seidenari S, Giusti F, Pepe P, Mantovani L. Contact Sensitization in 1094 Children Undergoing Patch Testing over a 7-year Period. Pediatric Dermatology. 2005; 22: 1-5.

Seidenari S, Manzini BM, Motolese A. Contact sensitization in infants: report of 3 cases. Contact Dermatitis. 1992; 27: 319-20.

Sevila A, Romaguera C, Vilaplana J, Botella R. Contact dermatitis in children. Contact Dermatitis. 1994; 30: 292-4.

Sfia M, Dhaoui MA, Doss N. Consort allergic dermatitis to cosmetic agents in a 10-year-old young girl. Contact Dermatitis. 2007; 57: 56-7.

Shah M, Lewis FM, Gawkrodger DJ. Patch testing in children and adolescents: five years' experience and follow-up. Journal of the American Academy of Dermatology. 1997; 37: 964-8.

Sharma VK, Asati DP. Pediatric contact dermatitis. Indian Journal of Dermatology, Venereology and Leprology. 2010; 76: 514-20.

Sidwell RU, Francis ND, Basarab T, Morar N. Vesicular Erythema Multiforme-like Reaction to Para-Phenylenediamine in a Henna Tattoo. Pediatric Dermatology. 2008; 25: 201-4.

Silverberg NB, Licht J, Friedler S, Sethi S, Laude T. Nickel Contact Hypersensitivity in Children. Pediatric Dermatology. 2002; 19: 110-3.

Smith WJ, Jacob SE. The role of allergic contact dermatitis in diaper dermatitis. Pediatric Dermatology. 2003; 26: 369-70.

Smith-Sivertsen T, Dotterud LK, Lung E. Nickel allergy and its relationship with local nickel pollution, ear piercing, and atopic dermatitis: A population-based study from Norway. Journal of the American Academy of Dermatology.1999; 40: 726-35.

Stables GI, Forsyth A, Lever RS. Patch testing in children. Contact Dermatitis. 1996; 34: 341-4.

Straus HW. Artificial Sensitization of Infants to Poison Ivy. Journal of Allergy. 1931; 2: 137-46.

Temesvari E, Racz I. Nickel sensitivity from dental prosthesis. Contact Dermatitis. 1988; 18: 50-1.

Uhr J, Dancis J, Ghantz Newmann C. Delayed Hypersensitivity in Premature Neonatal Humans. Nature. 1960; 187:1130-1.

Van Hoogstraten IMW, Andersen KE, Von Blombert BME, Boden D, Bruynzeel DP, Burrows D, et al. Reduced frequency of nickel allergy upon oral nickel contact at an early age. Clinical and Experimental Immunology. 1991; 85: 441-5.

Veien NK, Borchorst E, Hattel T, Laurberg G. Stomatitis or systemically-induced contact dermatitis from metal wire in orthodontic materials. Contact Dermatitis. 1994; 30: 210-3.

Veien NK, Hattel T, Justesen O, Norholm A. Contact dermatitis in children. Contact Dermatitis. 1982; 8: 373-5

Wantke F, Hemmer W, Jarisch R, Gotz M. Patch test reactions in children, adults and the elderly. A comparative study in patients with suspected allergic contact dermatitis. Contact Dermatitis. 1996; 34: 316-9.

Warshaw EM, Nelsen DD, Maibach HI, Marks JG, Zug KA, Taylor JS. Positive patch test reactions to lanolin: cross-sectional data from the North American contact dermatitis group, 1994 to 2006. Dermatitis. 2009; 20: 79-88.

Weston WL, Weston JA, Kinoshita J, Kloepfer S, Carreon L, Toth S, et al. Prevalence of positive epicutaneous tests among infants, children and adolescents. Pediatrics. 1986; 78: 1070-4.

Wilkowska A, Grubska-Suchanek E, Karwacka I, Szarmach H. Contact allergy in children. Cutis. 1996; 58: 176-80.

Wohrl S, Hemmer W, Focke M, Gotz M, Jarisch R. Patch Testing in Children, Adults, and the Elderly: Influence of Age and Sex on Sensitization Patterns. Pediatric Dermatology. 2003; 20: 119-23.

Wolf G, Hoger PH. Hypoallergenic and non-toxic emollient therapies for children. Journal der Deutschen Dermatologischen Gesellschaft. 2009; 7: 50-60.

Wolf R, Wolf D, Tuzun B, Tuzun Y. Diaper dermatitis. Clinics in Dermatology. 2000; 18: 657-660.

Worm M, Aberer W, Agathos M, Becker D, Brasch J, Fuchs T, et al. Patch testing in children - recommendations of the German Contact Dermatitis Research Group (DKG). Journal of the German Society of Dermatology. 2007; 5: 107-9.